OXFORD MEDICAL PUBLICATIONS

Arthritis and Rheumatism

THE FACTS

Arthritis and Rheumatism

THE FACTS

BY

J.T. SCOTT,

M.D., F.R.C.P.

Consultant Physician, Charing Cross Hospital, London; Honorary Physician, Kennedy Institute of Rheumatology

with an introduction by

DOROTHY EDÉN

OXFORD UNIVERSITY PRESS

Oxford New York Toronto Melbourne

OXFORD UNIVERSITY PRESS
Oxford London Glasgow
New York Toronto Melbourne
Nairobi Dar es Salaam Cape Town
Kuala Lumpur Singapore Hong Kong Tokyo
Delhi Bombay Calcutta Madras Karachi

and associate companies in
Beirut Berlin Ibadan Mexico City

First published by Oxford University Press, Oxford, 1980
First issued as an Oxford University Press paperback, 1981

British Library Cataloguing in Publication Data

Scott, J T

Arthritis and rheumatism.—(Oxford medical publications).
1. Arthritis 2. Rheumatism
I. Title II. Series
616.7′2 RC933 79-41660
ISBN 0-19-261168-2
ISBN 0-19-520278-3 pbk.
UK ISBN 0-19-286022-4 pbk.

This printing (last digit): 9 8 7 6 5 4 3 2 1
Printed in the United States of America

To all patients with rheumatic
diseases, who hopefully await
the progress of medical research,
this book is respectfully and
sympathetically dedicated.

Foreword

by

DOROTHY EDEN

novelist

Arthritis is a thorny word that seems to speak of pain. I myself, after twenty years of keeping rheumatoid arthritis at bay, call it a game of patience, of stoicism, of common sense, and, above all, of optimism.

The various forms of arthritis are all far too prevalent, and many of them have been with the human race for many thousands of years, at least as far as we can judge from ancient writings and archaelogical remains. The joint disease endured by a Roman Emperor in A.D. 68 was probably arthritis.

But much has been learned since those far-off days, even since the last century when rheumatism was the all-embracing definition of every ache and pain.

Dr Scott's scholarly book admirably sets out all that is known up to this time about the surprisingly large number of forms of arthritis, and the consequently differing treatments. He is honest about the lack of a cure, but has much to tell us about the alleviation of pain, and the slowing up of the depredations of the disease.

A cure will eventually be found, but I doubt that it will be one of the superstitious ones listed in Chapter 4. Arthritis is not only painful and at times frightening, but it is also intensely boring, an unwanted tenant in one's body that restricts so many activities. Reading that hopeful list of 'cures' may at least relieve a little of the boredom!

This is a book which will be invaluable to laymen, medical students, and doctors generally; the layman, especially the arthritic, is going to find Chapter 4 on methods of treatment, either by drugs or surgery, of particular interest. I can confirm that I have a successful record of drug treatment, and an outstandingly successful 'spare part' surgery record, having discarded one hip and two knees, operations that have rejuvenated my life.

Since rheumatoid arthritis and osteoarthrosis are the most prevalent forms of joint disease, the chapters on these will probably prove the most interesting, although the sad chapter on Still's disease is highly important. There are many other less-known and sometimes horrifying forms of arthritic diseases, such as those relating to haemophilia. I suppose that to call these diseases fascinating is hardly an apt description, but I do use it because this is not only an informative but a very readable book.

So I write this introduction from the other side of the fence, the patient who can vouch for the knowledge of the author. Dr Scott is a man of world-wide eminence in his field, and dedicated to finding the remaining elusive pieces of the puzzle of arthritis in all its forms. He is to be congratulated on this extremely useful and knowledgeable book.

Preface

'*Arthritis and rheumatism: the facts*' is intended to form a fitting companion to the other books in this series. Rheumatic diseases are widespread, often disabling, and rightly a matter of general concern. Although a few good books about them have been written for the public, and the Arthritis and Rheumatism Council produces excellent handbooks for patients, obtainable through family doctors, a larger number of other books are seriously misleading. I was therefore pleased to accept the invitation of the Oxford University Press to undertake what it is hoped will be a useful contribution to their series.

The primary purpose of this book is to provide a background of knowledge on the subject for the interested reader. Realizing that such a reader will only too often have first-hand acquaintance with one or other of the rheumatic diseases, either personally or in a close friend or relative, I hope to be the cause neither of unfounded optimism nor of unnecessary distress. Nothing written in the book is intended to replace proper consultation between patient and doctor. Here we can only discuss diseases: doctors treat people, which is a very different matter.

However, consultation time in our busy world tends to be limited and for patients under the care of their family practitioners the book will give supplementary information which can be studied at leisure. Others may also find it of value—nurses, physiotherapists, occupational therapists and other health workers, together with the growing number of laboratory scientists and technicians, not in themselves medical men and women, but whose work is closely concerned with some aspect of the rheumatic diseases and who wish to survey the whole subject briefly and in no great depth. It is even possible that medical students and doctors working in other fields may have some use for the book, but students should be warned that it does not contain enough to get them through M.B. finals! It is no substitute for text-books or reference works.

Preface

In the preparation of this book, and particularly the illustrations, I should like to express my thanks to members of the Departments of Medical Illustration and Physiotherapy at Charing Cross Hospital. I have also greatly appreciated the comments and guidance given to me by the publishers.

London J.T.S.

Contents

1

Background: The rheumatic diseases

Rheumatism is a common name for many aches and pains which have yet no peculiar appellation though owing to many different causes.

William Heberden (1710–1801)
Commentaries on the History and Cure of Disease

The words 'arthritis' and 'rheumatism' are everyday terms, usually used without a clear idea of their actual meaning or knowledge of their causes. Arthritis means simply inflammation of a joint, in the same way that appendicitis signifies inflammation of the appendix. To this extent it is an acceptable term, but on its own tells nothing of the cause or type of joint inflammation. It is therefore usually qualified by an adjective–for example, rubella arthritis is a trivial and transient pain and swelling of the joints which occasionally accompanies German measles; tuberculous arthritis (now rare in this country) occurs when a joint is infected by the tubercle bacillus; while rheumatoid arthritis refers to a chronic and sometimes disabling inflammation and destruction involving many of the joints of the body; we still know all too little of its causation. There are hundreds of other types of arthritis.

'Arthritis' is thus a definable term, though by itself an inadequate diagnostic label, but 'rheumatism' has no precise medical meaning at all. The word appears to have been introduced in medieval times to designate pain caused by a faulty flow of the cardinal humours of the body (blood, phlegm, choler, and melancholy), and is derived from the Greek words *rheuma* and *rheos* meaning a stream or flow (thus, in a more scientific context, a rheostat controls the flow of electricity). Gout, from the latin word *gutta*, meaning a drop, arose from the concept of a humour dripping into a joint cavity, particularly the joint at the base of the great toe. We no longer believe in these humours and modern physiology and pathology ignore their mystical combinations and fluxes. A physician can make a diagnosis of 'rheumatoid arthritis' or 'rheumatic fever' because such terminology, although based on an unsatisfactory and archaeic etymology, has come to be defined by scientically determined diagnostic criteria. The fact remains that 'rheumatism', although used as a generic name to cover all the rheumatic diseases, has in itself no diagnostic meaning whatsoever, with the exception that the term 'acute rheumatism' was understood until quite recently to refer to rheumatic fever.

The reader will already have begun to appreciate the difficulty of the physician, seeking honest and frank communication with his patient, who is confronted with the question: 'Do I have rheumatism, doctor?' I used to reply, 'I don't know what "rheumatism" is', until a long-suffering lady retorted: 'Well, you certainly would if you had it'. A patient who is told by his doctor that he has 'rheumatism' is quite justified in asking for a more precise definition of his problem.

Out of this confusion we can still talk of 'the rheumatic diseases', expert knowledge of which is required of the rheumatologist. Rheumatology has been broadly defined by the International League against Rheumatism as follows: 'Rheumatology is a branch of medicine concerned with a heterogeneous group of diseases and disorders commonly affecting the locomotor system. They may arise from primary pathological processes in connective tissue structures, from disorders of their function, or as a manifestation of systemic disease. Their common denominator appears to be involvement of connective tissue. Although joints appear to be the main site of symptoms, the arthritis is only one component of a constitutional illness of considerable complexity.' These disorders, which we will call the rheumatic diseases, thus comprise numerous derangements of the musculo-skeletal, articular (joint), and locomotor (movement) systems, with special reference to joint disease, except for those which are due to primary disease of the nerves of the body, which fall within the province of the neurologist.

History

Some of the rheumatic diseases have been recognized since ancient times, while others have been defined only relatively recently. A brief description of rheumatic fever appears in the works of Hippocrates (460-370 B.C.). In 1676 Thomas Sydenham, the greatest physician of his century, gave the first full description of acute rheumatic fever: 'It is commonest . . . during the autumn, chiefly attacking the young and vigorous–those in the flower of their age.' After a few days 'the patient is attacked by severe pain in the joints in turn, and affects the one that it attacks last with redness and swelling.' Sydenham also described involuntary, jerky muscle movements as chorea, or St. Vitus's dance, although he did not appreciate their association with rheumatic fever. Later physicians recognized the serious forms of heart disease which can result from rheumatic fever, which 'licks the joints and bites the heart'. We fortunately see little of rheumatic fever in developed countries nowadays but it is still a major problem in other parts of the world.

Gout is described in Hippocratic writings as 'the most violent, tenacious and painful of joint affections', and there is no doubt that this disorder too was well recognized by writers of classical times. Again it was Sydenham, himself a sufferer, who gave such a detailed and accurate clinical description of gout that it became possible to distinguish it from other types of arthritis. Gout appears to have been very common in England during the seventeenth and eighteenth centuries and there is a formidable list of eminent victims–monarchs, politicians, scientists, physicians, clerics, and men of letters. Satirical writers and caricaturists of those times did not fail to draw on such a rich source of material. In 1840 the Rev. Sydney Smith, Dean of St. Paul's, wrote: 'What a singular disease gout is; it seems as if the stomach fell down into the foot. The smallest deviation from the right diet is immediately punished by limping and lameness, and the innocent ankle and blameless instep are tortured for the vices of the nobler organs.'

The same period, however, saw the beginnings of scientific study of uric acid and its role in producing gout. During the nineteenth century Sir Alfred Garrod demonstrated that the blood of gouty subjects contained an excess of uric acid which became deposited in crystalline form in the joints. Developments in more recent years have included the realization that such an excess of uric acid may have different causes and, with appropriate drugs, a facility to control both the acute gouty attack and the level of the uric acid in the blood, thus transforming this painful and crippling scourge of the centuries into the most easily treatable of the rheumatic diseases.

As far as most of the other rheumatic diseases are concerned, however, it was only comparatively recently that medical writers began to draw any distinction between them, and today it is practically impossible to disentangle the old descriptions. It is, of course, readily understandable that physicians of former days, preoccupied as they were with the terrifying infections and epidemics which were then rampant, when men, women, and children died on the whole at a far younger age than they do today, had little opportunity or leisure to observe and study the chronic rheumatic diseases. Nevertheless, the absence of early clear descriptions of, for example, rheumatoid arthritis, a common inflammatory disease of joints with striking and characteristic clinical signs, is remarkable, and the intriguing possibility has been raised that the disease is one of comparatively recent times. A case has been made, however, for the Byzantine Emperor Constantine IX (A.D. 980–1055) being a victim; much earlier the historian Suetonius tells us that the hands and feet of the Roman Emperor Galba (A.D. 68–69) were severely deformed by '*articulari morbo*', which has been translated in the Loeb Classical Library as gout, but which could equally well refer to rheumatoid arthritis.

The first differentation of rheumatoid arthritis is usually attributed to Landré-Beauvais (1800), physician to the Saltpêtrière Hospital in Paris, but nomenclature remained completely confused. Garrod (1859) proposed the name rheumatoid arthritis. 'Although', he wrote, 'unwilling to add the number of names, I cannot help expressing a desire that one might be found for this disease . . . perhaps *rheumatoid arthritis* would answer the object, by which term I should wish to imply an inflammatory affection of the joints not unlike rheumatism [by which Garrod meant rheumatic fever] but differing materially from it.' The name became widely adopted. The modern era of intensive investigation into immunological aspects of rheumatoid arthritis may be said to have commenced with the discovery of an antibody called rheumatoid factor, detectable in the blood of most patients with rheumatoid arthritis, by the Norwegian immunologist Waaler in 1940. Since then a variety of immunological abnormalities have been found in rheumatoid arthritis and other inflammatory disorders of connective tissue, including constellations of antibodies reacting with various chemical components of the body. Some of these abnormalities may play a part in producing tissue damage, but underlying causes remain obscure. We shall return to this in later chapters.

Chronic arthritis, including rheumatoid arthritis, can occur in children, a fact appreciated by the paediatrician G. F. Still of Great Ormond Street Children's Hospital, in London, and the name 'Still's disease' is used to refer to a certain pattern of childhood arthritis.

Other types of joint inflammation can closely resemble rheumatoid arthritis both in their symptoms and in the appearance of the diseased tissues as seen under the microscope, but they are now known to be quite separate entities. For example, ankylosing spondylitis involves particularly the sacro-iliac joints at the base of the spine and the ligaments attached to the vertebrae, leading in advanced cases to rigidity ('poker back'). Evidence of ankylosing spondylitis has been found in ancient skeletons but the literature on the subject appears to start with an M. D. thesis written in 1691 by an Irishman called Bernard Connor, followed by several European descriptions in the last century. Related to ankylosing spondylitis are the types of arthritis which sometimes accompany infections of the genital tract and colon, and also the skin disease psoriasis.

The common condition nowadays known as osteoarthrosis, or osteoarthritis, has also been identified in the skeletons of prehistoric man and animals but again clinical recognition is a comparatively recent matter, although William Heberden (1710–1801) described the small nodes on the fingers which are a feature of generalized osteoarthrosis and which usually bear his name ('Heberden's nodes'): 'Digitorum Nodi. What are these little hard knobs, about the size of a small pea, which are frequently seen upon the fingers, particularly a little below the top near the joint? They have no connection with the gout, being found in persons who never had it; they continue for life; and being hardly ever attended by pain, or disposed to become sores, are rather unsightly than inconvenient, though they must be of some little hinderance to the use of the fingers.'

The term *malum coxae senilis* was devised by Adams of Dublin in 1857, referring to the type of osteoarthrosis which affects the hip joint alone, but the general distinction between rheumatoid arthritis and osteoarthrosis was clarified only during the present century.

So far we have been considering conditions where joints are the main site of symptoms, but many rheumatic disorders, some of them extremely common, affect other soft tissues of the locomotor system. They are sometimes referred to as 'non-articular rheumatic diseases'. Examples include the ubiquitous disorders of intervertebral discs. It is rather surprising that the features of prolapsed intervertebral discs were first described as recently as 1934 by Mixter and Barr in the U.S.A., although the syndromes* of sciatica and lumbago, of which disc injuries are important causes, have been recognized for centuries.

Generalized pains in the soft tissues of the body have been known by various names, such as 'muscular rheumatism' and 'fibrositis', a term proposed by Sir William Gowers in 1904, since he believed that the fibrous tissues were inflamed. Recent years have seen some progress in our understanding of the problem. It is recognized that a multiplicity of factors may precipitate pains of this nature, from minor trauma (the technical term for injury) and nerve irritation to complex inflammatory disorders of connective tissue. The syndrome known as polymyalgia rheumatica, sometimes accompanied by inflammation of arteries in the scalp, has been defined as a common cause of musculoskeletal pain in the elderly.

The development of rheumatology

Because many of the rheumatic diseases manifest themselves as chronic, painful disorders of the musculo-skeletal system, lacking, at least until recently, adequate methods of prevention and treatment, their victims, not unnaturally, have concerned themselves with such palliative and symptomatic forms of physical therapy as are to be found at spas and similar centres. Nor is this in itself necessarily to be condemned: whatever the short-comings of old-type cures and watering places, properly applied physical treatment, with its modern tendency towards self-reliance, often in a group environment, engenders a more positive

*Syndrome: from a Greek derivation meaning 'running together': a set of several associated signs and symptoms.

reaction to illness and disability than does the consumption of pills, and the morbidity and mortality of balneotherapy* (accidental or suicidal) is surely less than that of salicylates and other drugs which we prescribe so readily. Be that as it may, such forms of treatment had a considerable influence on the early development of rheumatology. In England in 1931, for example, the section of Balneology and Climatology of the Royal Society of Medicine joined with the Section of Electrotherapeutics to form the Section of Physical Medicine, which in 1973 became the Section of Rheumatology and Rehabilitation.

There have however been other influences, which can now be seen to have exerted a much more profound effect, such as the founding of academic departments (the first professorial Chair of Rheumatology in the United Kingdom was established at Manchester in 1953), which have contributed to the training of large numbers of rheumatologists throughout the world, besides stimulating research and setting exemplary standards of clinical practice. Within the framework of modern rheumatology have evolved many of the advances in clinical immunology and epidemiology, together with concepts of scientific clinical techniques such as the design of therapeutic trials and establishment of diagnostic criteria.

Along with these developments in the clinical field, national and international organizations have been established to initiate and coordinate the fight against the rheumatic diseases. The modern renaissance in these diseases and their prevention can be dated to papers such as Glover's (1927) 'Report on chronic rheumatism to the Ministry of Health', and to the formation of the Committee on Rheumatic Diseases by the Royal College of Physicians of London in 1935. This formed the nucleus of the Arthritis and Rheumatism Council, which today supports much of the research and education in rheumatic diseases, and to which the credit should be given for having made the Government and medical profession aware of the great social and industrial importance of this group of diseases in Great Britain. The British League against Rheumatism consists of scientific and community sections, representing the medical and other health profes-

*Treatment in baths.

sions, patients, and voluntary bodies. Affiliated organizations include the Arthritis and Rheumatism Council, the British Rheumatism and Arthritis Association (primarily concerned with patient welfare), and the Royal Association for Disability and Rehabilitation.

The International League against Rheumatism (ILAR) was formed in 1927, well before the present constituent regional leagues EULAR (European League against Rheumatism), PANLAR (Pan American League against Rheumatism), and SEAPAL (South-East Asia and Pacific Area League against Rheumatism). The original function of ILAR and the regional leagues was to organize international scientific congresses every four years, but as part of the new constitution of 1974 six co-ordinated standing committees were established:

1. *International and National Agencies*, co-ordinating ILAR's work with that of other international agencies and the World Health Organization.
2. *Education*, collecting data on education of rheumatologists and ancillary personnel and identifying areas where improvements can be made.
3. *Publications*, such as the ILAR *Handbook of Rheumatology* and any other publications issued with the authority of ILAR.
4. *Epidemiology*, studying rheumatic diseases in communities, nomenclature, and diagnostic criteria.
5. *International Clinical Studies*, co-ordinating clinical trials to avoid reduplication of research and setting reference centres on diagnostic criteria and laboratory tests, in collaboration with The World Health Organization.
6. *Social and Community Agencies*, developing parallel national, social, and community agencies responsible for fund-raising, research, patient welfare, education, and pressure on governmental departments to produce resources.

Social and economic aspects

The rheumatic diseases exact an enormous toll, both in individual misery and economic cost to the community. A detailed consideration of these aspects is beyond the scope of this book, but details of the situation in the United Kingdom are to be found in a recent report on problems and progress in health care for rheumatic disorders, based on evidence collected for presentation to the Royal Commission on the National Health Service. It is entitled *The challenge* *of arthritis and rheumatism* (1977)* and it should be consulted by anyone interested in the problem. The conclusions of the report are based on careful assessment of available data, and we can refer to them briefly in the next few pages.

Rheumatic diseases can occur at any age. Rheumatic fever is fortunately nowadays rare in developed countries (though still common in other parts of the world), but a variety of other rheumatic conditions is encountered in childhood and adolescence. The chances of acquiring some rheumatological disorder increase substantially with age—approximately 5 per cent of persons between the ages of 16 and 44 are affected, compared with 23 per cent of persons between 45 and 64, and 41 per cent of these aged 65 and over.

The prevalence of rheumatic disease varies with sex as well as with age. Rheumatoid arthritis, for example, is more common in women than in men, a tragic situation when the mother of a young family is affected, whereas other diseases, such as gout and ankylosing spondylitis, are much more frequent in men. Certain occupations carry their own particular risks, such as the high frequency of back troubles in miners or the various injuries of sportsmen.

The scope of the rheumatic diseases has already been outlined. In the working population they can be considered as three major groups of conditions:

1. *Arthritis*. Rheumatoid arthritis is the most disabling of rheumatic disorders, spells off work averaging ten months in men and twice this length in women. Osteoarthrosis is the other big cause identified specifically in incapacity data, the average spell lasting four months in men and over five months in women. As we have seen, there are many other forms of arthritis, naturally of great concern to individual patients, but numerically less important.

2. *Back pain*. Often, but by no means always, caused by intervertebral disc disease, this is an extremely common rheumatic condition and causes a similar amount of time lost from work.

3. *Other rheumatic problems*. These include many types of non-

*Edited by Dr. P.H.N. Wood and published by the British League against Rheumatism, c/o the Arthritis and Rheumatism Council, 8–10 Charing Cross Road, London WC2H 0HN, 94 pages, price 50 p (plus 10 p postage).

articular or soft tissue rheumatism (such as 'frozen shoulder' and polymyalgia rheumatica) as well as the less common but often serious conditions such as the diffuse inflammatory disorders of connective tissue.

It has been estimated that over eight million people in Great Britain will consult their general practitioner with some form of rheumatic problem during the course of a year, and that 23 per cent of patients seen by general practitioners have some sort of rheumatic complaint. Periods of absence from work average six weeks, leading to the overall loss of 44 million working days a year.

Services for patients

Rheumatic sufferers clearly require a wide range of general services—in primary care (general practice), from other health professionals (nurses, physiotherapists, occupational therapists, chiropodists, and social workers), and from specialist services (consultant physicians, rheumatologists, orthopaedic surgeons, rehabilitation physicians, and supporting services). It is again beyond the scope of this book to consider these matters in any detail: the overall situation is improving but still leaves a great deal to be desired.

The burden on the general practitioner is heavy. About one-fifth of his patients will consult him with some sort of rheumatic disorder. Yet many general practitioners have qualified with hardly any effective education about the diagnosis and management of rheumatic problems and will have learnt only through the hard grind of individual experience. Fortunately, owing in no small measure to the efforts of the Education Sub-committee of the Arthritis and Rheumatism Council, undergraduate medical training in rheumatology in the United Kingdom is now becoming more realistic: interest of the students in the intriguing niceties of immunopathology is sharpened by the knowledge that an awareness of these problems will be required in their final examinations. Apart from this, I am often touched by the spontaneous interest which the younger generation of students shows in our rheumatic patients and their personal problems, and the application of scientific methods in diagnosis and treatment.

Postgraduate and continuing education has also developed over the past few years and there is every opportunity for general practitioners to keep abreast with developments in medicine and surgery, including the rheumatic diseases. Certainly some general practitioners nowadays have an admirable knowledge of rheumatology, having developed a special expertise by their reading and experience, by attending courses, and by holding clinical assistantships in hospital clinics. Direct access to laboratory and radiological facilities is now available to most general practitioners; many practices have nurses and health visitors attached. We should be encouraging the further participation of general practitioners in the diagnosis and management of the rheumatic diseases: it is estimated that over a quarter of such patients referred to hospital could have been managed by the general practitioner himself, with consequent easing of the strain on the hospital services and shortening of waiting lists for outpatient attendance.

It is also estimated that there are about 500 qualified osteopaths and chiropractors and some 3000 unqualified persons earning their livelihood—sometimes handsomely—by offering treatment for rheumatic disorders in the United Kingdom. Some of these people are in fact skilful physiotherapists and many no doubt possess the ability to give helpful psychological support, but many of these unqualified practitioners are charlatans and their success is a poor reflection of the confidence of the public in our medical services in this field. However, there is again evidence that many available supporting services provided by the National Health Service and by local authorities are in fact under-utilized: contact with welfare and social services is often inadequate and facilities are insufficiently publicized.

A vast amount of support is indeed offered in the United Kingdom by some official agencies as well as by all sorts of voluntary and charitable bodies, not to mention countless admirable instances of individual effort. There is general awareness of the need to help physically handicapped people, and the range of services available includes industrial rehabilitation and retraining, practical assistance in the home, housing adaptation, the provision of aids and meals, recreational facilities, assistance with travelling and holidays, and other monetary grants and loans together with day residential care where necessary. Rheumatic sufferers have benefited over the years from the increasing attention and resources being directed to social service departments. However, we have little idea of the overall cost-effectiveness of these services: many have never been evaluated and it is known that there is a wide variation in their implementation by different local authorities. Further, the central collection of information by the Department of Health and Social Security is now related primarily to the degree of disability rather than to its cause, so that data relating specifically to rheumatic disorders are no longer readily available. About one-third of all disabled persons owe their disability to rheumatic diseases, the proportion rising with age.

Although many rheumatic illnesses can be dealt with quite adequately by general practitioners and their supporting facilities, further help is often required from hospital-based specialist services—for diagnostic consultation, for the supervision of complicated forms of drug treatment, for admission to hospital beds of more seriously ill patients, for medical or surgical assessment and treatment, and for specialized rheumatological rehabilitation. The rheumatologist is the physician who is responsible for such services. As with many other medical specialties, the work-pattern of rheumatologists varies to some extent. Some combine their work with wider interest in internal medicine, others practise 'pure rheumatology', while others can offer special mastery and experience in fields of medicine which are not exclusively related to the rheumatic diseases, such as general medical rehabilitation or clinical immunology. Each type of appointment has its own particular advantages depending to a large extent on local and individual circumstances and requirements, although some of us dislike the continued official designation, in many instances, of 'Rheumatology and Rehabilitation' as a single specialty. Of course the rheumatologist must be an expert in rehabilitation as it is relevant to his own patients, but there is no reason in general why he should be an authority, for example, on rehabilitation of people who have had a stroke or a heart attack, where the skills of the neurologist and the cardiologist are required. Whatever the emphasis of his interests, however, today's consultant rheumatologist in the United Kingdom is required to possess a higher medical qualification and to have undergone adequate training and experience both in general medicine and in the rheumatic diseases, according to criteria which have been laid down by the Royal College of Physicians.

Background: the rheumatic diseases

The past few years have seen an encouraging improvement in the numbers of consultant rheumatologists but there remains a considerable regional variation, with limited availability, for example, in Mersey, the South-West, west Midlands and Yorkshire: a number of area health authorities in England and Wales, responsible for several million people, still lack specialist advice in rheumatology. There is also an unsatisfactory variation in the availability of beds, waiting times for outpatient appointments, and supporting services such as occupational therapy.

Another major advance in the management of rheumatic diseases has been the application of orthopaedic surgery, the most important single example probably being the introduction of total hip replacement in osteoarthrosis, often dramatically transforming a pain-wracked cripple into a free-striding healthy man or woman. Surgery is also making an important impact in rheumatoid arthritis. Such developments—like those in other fields of medicine such as the treatment of kidney disease by dialysis or transplantation—could scarcely have been foreseen 20 or 30 years ago, and it is hardly the fault of doctors, administrators, or politicians that our resources are quite inadequate to deal effectively with the situation. The extent of these constraints is nevertheless disquieting: waiting-lists for hip replacement extend up to several years in some areas of the United Kingdom. The waiting list for major orthopaedic surgery to rheumatoid patients varies in different European countries. For example, a period of from two to six months for hip replacement is quoted for France whereas it is as much as from one to three years in Norway, as it is in the United Kingdom.

The root of the situation lies in the fact that many western nations are failing to generate enough wealth to pay for the necessary number of hospital beds, nurses, and anaesthetists which would be required to overcome the problem. In addition misguided administration can result in orthopaedic surgeons spending a large proportion of their time on non-operative out-patient drudgery, often of a minor nature.

2

Connective tissue and joints

We have seen that rheumatology is concerned with disorders involving connective tissue and joints, and before going on to consider some of the more important rheumatic diseases–the main purpose of this book–we should perhaps give a brief and simple account of these tissues and structures. For a more detailed discussion the reader may wish to consult one of the standard modern textbooks on the rheumatic diseases.*

There are four main types of substance or tissue in the body: (1) epithelium, which provides a covering for the internal and external body surfaces, such as skin, intestine, and glandular tissues; (2) muscle; (3) nervous tissue; and (4) connective tissue. Connective tissue in general forms the framework of the body, including the skeleton. It comprises areolar tissue, the packing material of the body, together with more organized structures such as ligaments, cartilage, and bone. Where body movement is necessary, adjacent skeletal units articulate at specialized connective tissue zones that act as joints.

Like all body tissues, connective tissue is composed of individual parent units called cells, which produce various types of material (matrix) lying between the cells–intercellular fibres and ground substance. Connective tissue is characterized by a relatively large amount of this intercellular matrix. Various types of cell are found in connective tissue. These have different functions such as the production of proteins and other substances which constitute the intercellular matrix; the production of the various components of cartilage (these cells are called chondrocytes) and the formation and metabolism of bone; cells which have the capacity of engulfing and eliminating worn-out cells and debris or various types of foreign material; fat cells; and

*e.g. *Copeman's Textbook of the rheumatic diseases*, fifth edn (edited J.T. Scott). Churchill Livingstone, Edinburgh, London and New York (1978).
An introduction to clinical rheumatology, second edn (edited R.M. Mason and H.L.F. Currey). Pitman Medical Publishers, Tunbridge Wells (1975).

synovial cells, which form the lining layer of joints. Synovial cells produce synovial fluid which plays a part in the lubrication of joints and which provides substances necessary for the nutrition of chondrocytes in joint cartilage. Synovial cells can also swallow damaged tissue fragments or foreign material that has gained access to the joint.

The intercellular matrix consists of different types of fibres and ground substance. One of the important forms of fibre is called collagen, a protein of high tensile strength lying outside the cells and forming a constituent of skin, tendons, ligaments, cartilage, and bone. The inflammatory disorders of connective tissue (Chapter 10) were for a time known as 'collagen diseases' in the mistaken belief that the underlying cause lay in a derangement of collagen. This is not now believed to be the case and the term 'collagen disease' has been largely discarded. Elastic fibres are characterized by their extensibility and ability to resist deformation without being damaged: they therefore form an essential part of such structures as arteries, which pulsate with each beat of the heart, and some types of cartilage which also possess the property of recoiling after bending or stretching.

The ground substance of connective tissue is the material which lies between the cells and fibres. Its principal component is a family of very large molecules called proteoglycans, which consist essentially of a central core with numerous side-chains. Such a molecular structure is favourable to lubrication and protection against impact loading and vibration, as opposed to the tensile strength and rigidity provided by collagen. The past few years have seen a rapid advance in our knowledge of these various components of connective tissue and the biochemical anormalities which can occur in disease.

A lot of connective tissue is widely distributed and 'loose', serving an unspecialized flexible supporting and packing function, with many cells, much ground substance but few fibres. 'Compact' connective tissue is formed where strength rather than flexibility is the prime requirement, as in tendons and ligaments; here we find a great deal of collagen but little in the way of cells and ground substance. In bone, the strength is greatly increased by the deposition of insoluble calcium salts impregnating a network of collagen fibres. Compact connective tissue is differentiated into many important structures of the locomotor system. The fibrous capsules of joints are attached to the opposing bone ends and have a protective function. Ligaments are localized thickenings of a joint capsule forming strong and stabilizing attachments between bones. Tendons are similar structures attaching muscle to bone.

Cartilage is a very firm type of connective tissue composed of chrondrocytes lying in an abundant matrix, but without the mineral content of bone. According to its distribution, constitution, and function several types are described. These include:

1. Hyaline cartilage (Latin *hyalinus* = glass) a layer of which is found over the articular (Latin *artus* = joint) surfaces of bone where they form joints, as described below. Hyaline cartilage can withstand the immense loads to which the joints of the body are subjected. When a load is applied the cartilage is immediately deformed owing to the elasticity of its fibre-reinforced gel, followed by squeezing-out of fluid: when the load is removed there is immediate recovery followed by the flow of fluid back into the loaded area.

2. Fibrocartilage, which contains dense fibrous bundles. Fibrocartilage forms an important part of structures such as the intervertebral disc, which will be described below. Menisci are crescent-shaped pieces of fibrocartilage lying within some of the joints, notably the knee. They are liable to damage following injury, and are removed by the orthopaedic surgeon when the soccer-player has a 'cartilage operation' on his knee.

3. Yellow elastic cartilage is found in the cartilage of the ear-lobes and larynx.

Muscular contraction, transmitted through tendons, acts upon bone to produce movement which is facilitated by joints. The detailed anatomical description of the many different types of joint need not concern us. Two basic types are recognized: synovial* (or

*The origin of the term 'synovial' is obscure. '*Synovia*' is a late Latin term which appears to have been coined by the mediaeval physician Paracelcus to apply to the viscid 'egg-like' joint fluid (Latin *ovum* = egg). The word 'synovia' is sometimes used by medical writers, who should know better, to apply to synovial membranes. For this reason the word is better avoided; we can speak instead of 'synovial fluid' or 'synovial membrane'.

diarthrodial) joints, where there is a joint 'cavity' (containing synovial fluid) and free movement, as in limb-joints such as the knee or wrist; and synarthroses, where there is union between bones–fibrous or cartilagenous–without a joint cavity. The mobile synovial joints are involved in many of the rheumatic diseases, so an understanding of their basic anatomy is required. The most important example of a synarthrosis, from the clinical point of view, is the intervertebral disc.

Synovial joints are subdivided into many anatomical varieties, a detailed consideration of which is again unnecessary for our present purpose. Their basic structure is shown in Fig. 1. The two opposing bone ends (articular surfaces) are covered by a layer of hyaline articular cartilage. The fibrous joint capsule is attached near to the articular margin of the bones. The surface of the interior of the joint, except for that covered by cartilage, is lined by the delicate synovial membrane, which secretes synovial fluid into the joint cavity. Normally, only a minute amount of synovial fluid is formed, but excessive amounts (effusions) accumulate in various forms of arthritis. Tendons and ligaments also enter into the structure of joints, together, in some instances, with fibro-cartilagenous menisci, as already described. It should also be pointed out that synovial membrane lines not only

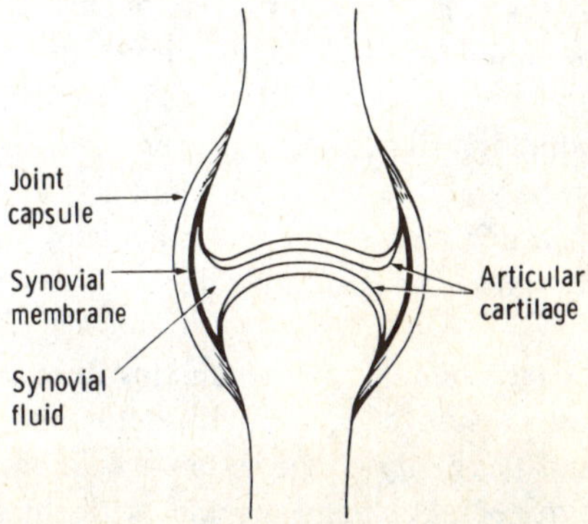

Fig. 1. Diagram of a typical synovial joint.

the joints themselves but also (a) the sheaths which protect tendons and (b) other sacs (bursae) which may or may not be directly connected with the joint cavity. Inflammation of synovial membrane in these situations is termed 'tenosynovitis' and 'bursitis' (see Chapter 11).

Human joints are incredibly efficient by engineering standards: the coefficient of friction is far lower than that of any non-biological system yet devised. Theories about joint lubrication have been vigorously debated. They are beyond the scope of our present discussion, but there appears little doubt that different forms of lubrication are of critical importance under different operating conditions–that is, when loads are light or heavy, gradual or sudden. There is also no doubt that the efficiency of joints is dependent upon a complex physico-chemical interrelationship of synovial fluid, synovial membrane, and healthy articular cartilage. The idea that impaired joint function can be restored by the injection of some form of synthetic lubricating fluid, like oiling a rusty hinge, is impossibly naive.

Let us finally consider our example of the second basic type of joint, the synarthrosis: the intervertebral disc, derangements of which (discussed in Chapter 11) are responsible for a great deal of pain and discomfort which most of us have experienced at one time or another. The main joints between the vertebral bodies–the bones of the back–are formed by intervertebral discs that have a unique connective tissue structure. They consist of fibro-cartilagenous plates which unite adjacent vertebrae (Fig. 2). The outer layers of this plate are formed of dense concentric bundles of collagen fibres, the annulus fibrosus. The orientation of these bundles is less well-defined behind, and their strength correspondingly less, than elsewhere, and the posterior longitudinal ligament behind the vertebral column is also relatively weak postero-laterally, which means that the spinal cord and its nerve roots lying within the spinal canal are vulnerable to pressure effects from disc disease.

Within the collagen bundles of the annulus fibrosus lies the nucleus pulposus, a softer portion of entirely distinct connective tissue which gives elasticity and flexibility to the vertebral column. The longitudinal ligaments of the vertebral column, together with the outer parts of the annulus fibrosus, are supplied with pain-sensitive nerves. Ageing and biochemical alterations may combine with mechanical stresses to

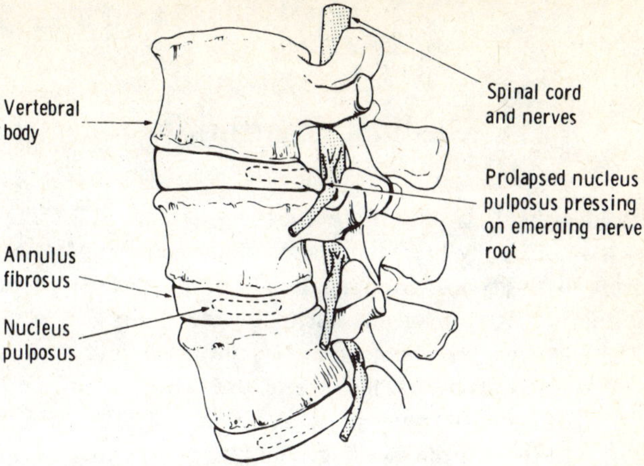

Fig. 2. Diagram of vertebrae and intervertebral discs. In the upper disc the nucleus pulposis has prolapsed backwards, pressing on an emerging nerve root.

cause protrusion of part of the nucleus pulposus through the weak parts of the annulus fibrosus and posterior longitudinal ligament.

So much, then, in these two opening chapters, for our background to rheumatology and the rheumatic diseases. We have not yet touched upon the pathological mechanisms–genetic, immunological, and biochemical–which are responsible for their causation and manifestations. These will be considered individually in the chapters that follow.

3

Rheumatoid arthritis

Rheumatoid arthritis is one of the most important of the rheumatic diseases. It is relatively common and in its more serious forms it can cause severe disability and crippling. It is a chronic disorder, developing over months or years, involving essentially the synovial joints of the body. The synovial membrane becomes inflamed and swollen, and infiltrated by inflammatory cells (see Plate 1). Because of the inflammation the amount of synovial fluid within the joint is increased, contributing further to the swelling. The inflamed synovial membrane is thrown up into folds called villi: it also extends over the surface of the articular cartilage forming a mass of tissue called a pannus, which burrows into the cartilage and underlying bone to produce the 'erosions' which are a characteristic feature of the disease (Fig. 3). The bone surfaces may stick together, leading to restricted movement, and weakness of associated ligaments and tendons contributes further to instability and partial dislocation of the joint.

Although basically a disease of joints, rheumatoid arthritis also

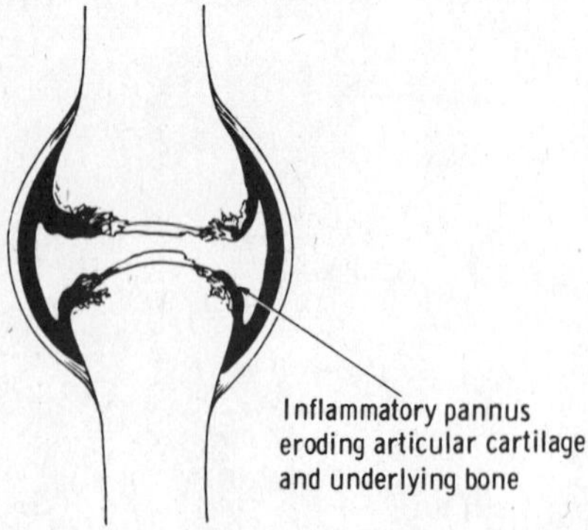

Fig. 3. Diagram of a rheumatoid erosion.

manifests itself in many other tissues. Characteristic 'nodules' are found under the skin in various situations, especially over the elbows, and in many internal organs, together occasionally with inflammation of the blood vessels (vasculitis). Different combinations of nodule formation and vasculitis can involve the skin (producing ulceration) and organs as widespread as the eye, heart, lungs, and nervous system. Added to this may be the general features of inflammation–fever, anaemia, and weight loss.

The disease can first manifest itself in various ways and its onset may be insidious or rapid. In one case pain and stiffness come on slowly and it is a matter of days or weeks before it is realized that anything serious is wrong. In another case the patient may feel quite well on retiring to bed only to awaken the next morning with painful swelling of one or several joints. Curiously enough, people with this more acute type of onset often fare better eventually than those in whom the process starts more slowly. Few or many joints become involved: in its characteristic form rheumatoid arthritis tends to be symmetrical in distribution, attacking particularly the joints of the hands (see Plate 2(a)), wrists, knees, and feet, but the pattern is quite variable. Later deformities include characteristic deviation and distortion of the fingers, hands, feet, and limbs. The joint affliction is set against a background, to a greater or lesser degree, of general ill-health: 'morning stiffness' is a striking and distressing symptom, several hours elapsing before the patient becomes mobile.

Rheumatoid arthritis is as variable in its course as in its distribution. It is often a disorder of 'exacerbations' and 'remissions', that is to say flares of disease activity punctuated by periods of respite. While it is unfortunately true that progression to serious deformity can occur, and that for things to 'burn themselves out' completely is not as common as one would wish, nevertheless with correct modern management the majority of sufferers can be kept from serious trouble and can continue to lead happy, active, and useful lives, albeit with a good deal of determination on their part. We shall have much more to say about treatment later.

Diagnosis

A patient coming to the doctor with early rheumatoid arthritis may pose quite a difficult problem in diagnosis, for there are many other possible causes of inflammatory arthritis, many of them fortunately benign. For example, a number of known viruses, such as rubella (German measles) can cause an arthritis which invariably clears completely after a period of days or weeks, and there are numerous other types of joint disease, some of them considered later in this book, which can resemble rheumatoid arthritis in its early stages. The physician may be able to reach a diagnosis as an immediate result of his examination–the discovery of rheumatoid nodules, for example, may be an important clue. X-rays of the joints may help, but are of limited usefulness in the very early stages, rheumatoid erosions rarely being visible until the disease has been present for more than three months.

Persons with suspected rheumatoid arthritis are always anxious to know what the 'blood tests' show. The doctor will certainly want to know the result of a routine blood cell count for various reasons, including the detection of anaemia. He will also request an erythrocyte sedimentation rate (E.S.R.). This is a simple and useful test which gives some idea of the degree of inflammation present. A column of blood, treated with an anticoagulant to prevent it clotting, is drawn up into a narrow vertical glass tube and the rate of sedimentation of the red cells in the plasma is observed. Normally there are only a few millimetres of clear plasma at the top of the column after a one-hour period, but inflammatory diseases produce changes in the proteins of the blood plasma which alter its viscosity, thus allowing the red cells to fall more rapidly. In some laboratories the plasma viscosity is measured directly instead: the same sort of information is obtained. The purpose of this test is to establish whether or not some inflammatory disorder is present (and also, if so, to follow its progress). Thus it is usually abnormal in rheumatoid arthritis, but normal in osteoarthrosis, which is not primarily an inflammatory disease. Beyond this it is of no specific diagnostic value–it tells nothing about the *type* of inflammation.

Blood may also be examined for the presence of 'rheumatoid factor'. This is a large molecular weight protein, mostly in the so-called IgM fraction, which acts as an antibody to, and reacts with, another fraction of protein called IgG. Proteins of this type, which are closely concerned with the body's immunological reactions, are called 'immunoglobulins'. The discovery of rheumatoid factor nearly 40 years ago was of very great theoretical interest with regard to our concept of immunological processes in rheumatoid arthritis. It also came to be of vital importance in classifying the types of arthritis in which rheumatoid factor is absent–'seronegative' arthritis as opposed to 'seropositive' rheumatoid disease. Unfortunately, in the individual patient, the test may not be all that helpful, being positive in only about 70 per cent of patients with rheumatoid arthritis, and tending to be negative in early or mild cases–that is, just the sort of patient where diagnostic help is required. Further, the test is by no means specific–that is to say it can be positive in other diseases, and indeed is so in a small proportion of the normal healthy population. With these qualifications, examination of the blood for rheumatoid factor can sometimes be a useful diagnostic test, and a high concentration to some extent indicates a rather poor outlook (prognosis); but careful interpretation of results is essential. The patient with little the matter with him, but who has been told this test has been positive, takes a lot of reassuring.

Other tests need not concern us. We should perhaps mention the difficulties when rheumatoid arthritis arises, as it may, in a single joint such as one knee. Now there are many other causes of inflammation of a single joint, such as bacterial infections which might require antibiotic treatment. It is sometimes necessary in these circumstances to withdraw some synovial fluid with a syringe and needle for bacteriological examination, or occasionally to take a small piece of synovial membrane for examination under the miscroscope. This procedure (biopsy) is usually done with a needle, or by direct visualization of the interior of the joint using an instrument called an arthroscope (Plate 3).

Who gets rheumatoid arthritis?

Rheumatoid arthritis appears to be widely distributed throughout all countries of the world. Estimates of its prevalence vary to some extent with the diagnostic criteria and epidemiological techniques employed. It is unquestionably a common disease: its overall frequency appears to be in the order of 1 per cent of the population. There may well be true regional variations. For example, some evidence from South Africa suggests that the frequency of occurrence may increase with a transition from rural to urban living, which if correct is an intriguing observation. The prevalence of the disease in certain tribes of native Africans was found to be 0.87 per cent: among the same people who had moved to an urban environment it was 3.3 per cent, much the same figure as for Europeans living in Africa. Disease in the rural Africans also tended to be milder. However, rheumatoid arthritis is found in town and rural communities in this country and elsewhere.

Contrary to popular belief, climate has little importance: it is true that some patients prefer warm or dry weather, and factors such as temperature and humidity may well have an effect on pain threshold, but there is no evidence that climate directly influences the occurrence or progress of rheumatoid arthritis, which is indeed found in all climatic conditions, temperate or tropical.

The onset of the disease can occur at any age, from infancy onwards, but most commonly between the ages of 30 and 60. Women are afflicted more frequently than men in a proportion of about two or three to one.

Strong familial clustering, as occurs in some of the other rheumatic diseases such as gout and ankylosing spondylitis, is not found in rheumatoid arthritis. During the last year or two information has been gathering about inherited genetic factors which influence susceptibility, and these may be of importance in some patients. We are still rather ignorant about this part of the problem, but overall there does not appear to be a strong hereditary aspect, a point of great importance to the young married woman with rheumatoid arthritis. Whatever the desirability of limiting the size of her family because of the physical strain which any large young family of children puts upon any mother, she need have little fear that the disease will appear in her offspring.

Can mental or physical stress have any bearing on the development of rheumatoid arthritis? Most of us like to seek cause and effect in the events of our lives and there are occasional patients with rheumatoid disease who confidently date the onset of their condition from an emotional shock or some other disturbance. Despite attempts to investigate the matter there remains no firm evidence that stress of this type causes rheumatoid arthritis, and my own feeling is that such associations are coincidental. It has been fashionable to describe rheumatoid arthritis as a psychosomatic disorder, and to delineate certain psychological types of person who are liable to develop the disease, but none of this is at all convincing. Of course, depression and frustration may follow in the wake of any chronic disabling disease. Indeed, it is remarkable how so many patients with rheumatoid arthritis maintain a cheerful disposition. On the other hand, a person's character can well influence the pattern of joint disease and the appearance of the articular erosions. Look at the deep, punched-out erosions in Plate 4. Such lesions, as was first pointed out by Prof. E. G. L. Bywaters, are seen in patients, usually men, who have a high pain threshold and who carry on with their normal physical activity: they often claim that they have never lost a day's work. Their bones remain well calcified because of constant use and the deep erosions are probably caused by movements of the limbs repeatedly raising the pressure within the joints, driving synovial fluid and debris through the damaged articular cartilage down into the ends of the bone. By contrast, other patients with low pain thresholds, who often make little effort to keep going, develop shallow erosions and decalcified bone (Plate 5). These patients are more often women.

Physical stress and trauma (or injury) are also sometimes claimed to predispose to the development of rheumatoid arthritis, but again there is no good evidence that they do so: this is occasionally a point of medico-legal importance, when rheumatoid arthritis comes on after some sort of injury for which compensation is being claimed. In such cases the relationship is again probably coincidental rather than causal. The situation sometimes arises, however, when injury is sustained to a particular joint and the pain and swelling fail to subside as expected. A little later signs of generalized rheumatoid arthritis appear, with predominant involvement of the joint which has been injured (Plate 6). To this extent trauma can exacerbate local joint damage in a patient in whom rheumatoid arthritis is developing: but this is not the same thing as saying that injury is actually causing rheumatoid arthritis.

The cause of rheumatoid arthritis

What then is the causative agent, or agents? The simple answer is that we do not yet know, although recent years have seen considerable advances in our understanding of the mechanisms whereby joints and other tissues become damaged in this disease.

There has been no shortage of theories. Suggestions have included some form of metabolic error (as occurs for example in diabetes or gout), dietary deficiency, an inbalance in the functions of the nervous system and an abnormality in endocrine or hormonal activity, the last idea receiving some initial support when it was discovered in 1949 that the acute signs and symptoms of rheumatoid arthritis responded dramatically to large doses of extracts of adrenal glands (cortisone). The theory of 'focal sepsis' held sway for many years. I think that physicians in the earlier part of the century can have had no clear understanding of the difference between rheumatic fever and rheumatoid arthritis; rheumatic fever had been shown to follow streptococcal tonsillitis (Chapter 8), so it must have seemed logical at the time to treat rheumatoid arthritis by removing any tissue or organ of the body where infection might conceivably lurk. At all events, countless teeth, tonsils, gall-bladders, and wombs were extirpated in the hope of amelioration—but all in vain.

The age of immunology was ushered in, as we have already seen, by the discovery of rheumatoid factor in 1940. MacFarlane Burnet, the Australian immunologist, published his hypothesis regarding 'self' and 'non-self' antigens in 1959, and the concept became popular that rheumatoid arthritis was an 'autoimmune' disease, implying an abnormal immune reaction directed against some body component—as if the body, which normally fights an invading organism like typhoid or tuberculosis, turned its attack on its own tissues. The problem is in fact much more complicated than this, but there is no doubt that immunological processes are closely concerned with the tissue damage which occurs in rheumatoid arthritis. It is well recognized that immune reactions, which have evolved and been retained because of their survival value in protecting the host against foreign invaders, can on occasion prove injurious to the host.

Evidence for immunological involvement in rheumatoid arthritis can be summarized thus:

1. The pannus of inflamed tissue growing from the synovial membrane contains a high proportion of lymphocytes and plasma

cells, types of blood cell which are known to be concerned in various stages of the immunological response. There are several types of lymphocyte, including so-called 'B lymphocytes' and 'T lymphocytes'.

2. There is abundant evidence of antigen–antibody activity in rheumatoid arthritis. An antigen is a substance, normally foreign to the host, which can elicit an immunological response, with or without accompanying inflammation. One form of response consists of the production, by B lymphocytes, of specific antibodies, which can react or combine with antigens. Immunological reactions of this type, traditionally concerned with the neutralization of antigens from harmful organisms, can involve antigens partially or wholly derived from host tissue, the concept of autoimmunity already mentioned. Molecular complexes of antigen combined with antibody can be detected by many different methods; they can be found in joint effusions from patients with rheumatoid arthritis, and have also been demonstrated in synovial membrane. In some patients, particularly those with widespread vasculitis, antigen–antibody complexes appear in the circulating blood. As we have seen, rheumatoid factor behaves as an antibody directed against IgG immunoglobulin, and can itself therefore be a constituent of antigen–antibody complexes. Antibodies directed against other host components, such as constituents of cell nuclei, characteristically found in systemic lupus erythematosus (Chapter 10), sometimes make their appearance in rheumatoid arthritis.

3. The combination of an antigen with its specific antibody also involves the activation and consumption of 'complement', which becomes incorporated in the antigen–antibody complex. Complement consists of a number of different proteins which are formed in sequence once the process of activation commences: some of them are capable of causing inflammation. Reduced levels of the proteins that make up complement are found in the synovial fluid of rheumatoid arthritics, indicating that they have been used up in complex-formation.

4. There are other types of immune response besides the classical antigen–antibody reaction (humoral immunity). One is called cell-mediated immunity involving the direct interaction of antigen and T lymphocytes. An indication of this type of response is the production by lymphocytes of substances called lymphokines: lymphokines are detectable in rheumatoid joints.

5. Other clinical conditions caused by abnormal immunological

reactivity, too complicated to describe in detail, may be associated with rheumatoid arthritis. These include Sjogren's syndrome, in which dryness of the mucous membranes of the eyes and enlargement of the salivary glands are combined with the presence of several auto-antibodies; Felty's syndrome, where the spleen is enlarged and the numbers of white cells in the blood reduced; and amyloid disease, where an abnormal protein fibril is deposited in the kidney and elsewhere, the latter, incidentally, being one of the rare causes of fatality in rheumatoid disease.

6. It is possible to suppress the immune response, either by the use of certain drugs or by other techniques which can reduce the number of lymphocytes and their products in the body. There is good evidence that such immunosuppression can reduce the activity of the rheumatoid inflammatory process, at least temporarily. Moreover, it is possible to remove circulating antigen–antibody complexes by specialized (and still largely experimental) methods known as plasmapheresis and it has been claimed that this is followed by transient improvement, particularly in those aspects of the disease which are unrelated to the joints themselves.

From considerations such as these there is no doubt that rheumatoid arthritis is a disease characterized by a good deal of immunological reactivity, and current theory ascribes many of the damaging processes of the disease to such reactions. It is envisaged that immune complexes in joint fluid attract white blood cells, the function of which is to engulf them. This process of phagocytosis is accompanied by the release of substances (enzymes) which can provoke an inflammatory response. Other contributing factors include the activation of complement and the process of cell-mediated immunity. It also appears probable that circulating immune complexes are associated with vasculitis and other signs of the disease not actually related to the joints.

Much has also been learnt about the manner in which the inflammatory pannus, growing from the inflamed synovial membrane, attacks and damages the cartilage and bone of the joint, and a number of enzymes have been isolated from rheumatoid synovial cells which are capable of destroying collagen fibres and proteoglycans, thus producing the more permanent ravages of the disease.

From what has been written the reader will, it is hoped, have seen that research work of the past few decades has revealed much of the processes and mechanisms of rheumatoid inflammation, but that basic questions remain to be answered. Why are some joints involved and not others? Why does the process of inflammation usually continue in a chronic manner over the years? Above all, if antigen–antibody reactions are so important, what is the actual nature of the antigen and why is it present?

The sustained nature of the immunological process in rheumatoid arthritis points to the continued presence of a stimulating antigen: the most likely source of such an antigen would, it is argued, be some form of infecting agent. The search for such an agent has been intensive but to date unavailing. Several claims have been made for the isolation of different varieties of bacteria from rheumatoid synovial membranes, but none has become accepted as a causative organism. Similar isolates have been obtained from non-rheumatoid joints, and they may represent merely the presence of 'passengers', not themselves producing the disease. Attempts to incriminate viruses have been similarly unsuccessful, either by direct culture from synovial membrane or from the study of circulating virus antibodies.

Rheumatoid arthritis has been called by the American rheumatologist Morris Ziff the 'immaculate infection'. Nevertheless the complexities of host–organism relationships in chronic viral infection continue to be studied by new and sophisticated techniques, and the possibility that rheumatoid arthritis represents an immunological reaction, in susceptible individuals, to infection by one or many different types of virus has by no means been discarded.

4

The treatment of rheumatoid arthritis

We cannot yet, unfortunately, speak in terms of either the prevention or cure of rheumatoid arthritis. We know little of its causes and how to counteract them. Much has nevertheless been learnt about the disease over the past few decades: standards of management have greatly improved, and while in a few cases the disease progresses inexorably despite all therapeutic efforts, most patients can be helped to lead useful and self-reliant lives.

As we have seen, rheumatoid arthritis is a chronic disease often characterized by periods of activity and quiescence. Sometimes it goes into complete remission, a fact for which we can be thankful but which makes therapeutic evaluation extremely difficult. If such clinical improvement should happen to take place, as it often does, while a patient is taking a certain diet, or wearing a copper bangle, or receiving acupuncture, it is only natural that the benefit should be attributed to the diet and so on: only the physician, who sees numerous other cases who have *not* responded to such treatment, realizes that the association is probably one of chance rather than one of cause and effect. Indeed for the same reason it is often difficult for the physician himself to assess the results of any form of treatment he has prescribed, and we have come to realize the necessity of the controlled clinical trial. In such a trial the progress of two identical groups of patients, only one of which is receiving the treatment under investigation, is carefully compared, preferably under 'double-blind' conditions, that is to say where neither the doctor nor the patient, during the progress of the trial, knows whether or not the treatment is being given in any particular instance. Of course careful attention has to be paid to the often difficult statistical and ethical problems inherent in this type of research.

Most of the drugs used in the rheumatic diseases have now been subjected to such evaluation, upon which to a large extent depends their acceptance by the medical profession. For example, gold salts were introduced for the treatment of rheumatoid arthritis as long ago as 1929: it soon became realized that they were probably effective and certainly occasionally toxic, but it was only after controlled trials, such as that carried out by the Empire Rheumatism Council and published in 1961, that the use of gold was properly evaluated. Nowadays any new drug is soon subjected to such critical investigation, without which no claims for any sort of therapeutic benefit can be readily accepted.

Generalization about the management of rheumatoid arthritis is impossible because no two patients are quite alike and the needs of one are different from those of another. In one instance widespread active inflammatory disease involving many joints, accompanied by constitutional features such as weight loss, fever, and anaemia, demands a period of rest and the introduction of appropriate drugs designed to bring the inflammation under control as far as possible. In another case progressive damage and deformity may be restricted to one or two joints, so that the question of local treatment, perhaps surgical, has to be considered. In yet another case it may be non-articular problems, such as vasculitis, rather than the joints themselves which require attention.

Subject to such reservations it is possible to consider the management of rheumatoid arthritis under five general headings:

1 Assessment and explanation.
2 Physical treatment.
3 Drugs.
4 Surgery.
5 Rehabilitation.

Assessment and explanation

It goes without saying that a proper diagnosis and assessment of function are necessary, as with any other medical condition. They can be undertaken by the patient's general practitioner, although in all but the mildest of cases it is as well to have a confirmatory opinion from a consultant rheumatologist, whose work has been described in Chapter 1. The extent to which hospital-based collaboration is thereafter necessary depends on the severity or complexity of the individual problem.

There can be no doubt about the desirability of a frank and full discussion between the doctor and patient. Those who attempt to acquire an intelligent understanding of their disease, as far as is possible where so much remains unknown, tend to do better in the long run—hence this book. Depression and anxiety are natural reactions on hearing the diagnosis, but there are real reasons for encouragement. Many victims of this disease fear that they may eventually have to spend their days in a wheelchair, and it cannot be too firmly stressed that with proper care this unhappy state is the lot of only a very few. It is difficult, particularly early in the disease, to answer questions about the outlook in any individual case, although some favourable and unfavourable features, mentioned in the previous chapter, have been identified. Surveys indicate quite definitely that only a minority of patients—even those whose disease is bad enough to warrant referral to a hospital department—are destined for severe disability. This must be brought home clearly and emphatically.

What else will the patient want to know? He—or rather she, for as we have already seen this disease is significantly more common in women than in men—she, then, will want to know what she can do to help herself, to 'fight the disease'. Well, the disease cannot be 'fought' just like that, but the patient who can surmount her problems with a buoyant attitude, practising assiduously, for example, the physical methods of treatment discussed below, will do well.

Many people ask their doctor about the effects of climate, which is probably of little importance, as discussed in the previous chapter, or whether any alteration of diet is necessary. As far as is known, rheumatoid arthritis is not caused by any dietary deficiency or imbalance. Claims have been made for treatment with special foodstuffs and metabolic treatments—vegetarian diets, vitamins, cod-liver oil, the Liefmann method, Dr. Dong's diet and so on, but none of these have been shown by any form of scientific evaluation to alter the course of the disease or its symptoms. To this extent, therefore, diet has no known part in the prevention or management of rheumatoid arthritis. Two special points should, however, be mentioned. In the first place, although diet is not considered to play a causative role in the development of the disease, it is important that the rheumatoid sufferer takes a properly balanced diet with an adequate supply of protein and vitamins; there is clear evidence that many patients fail to do so, either because of financial hardship or because sheer physical disability hinders shopping, cooking, and the preparation of meals. A study from Bristol some years ago showed how bread and butter and cups of tea could become a staple diet, with consequent anaemia due to lack of iron and other nutritional deficiencies. The patient, her family, and her physician must be alive to this possibility. Secondly, although severe active rheumatoid arthritis may be attended by loss of weight, this is by no means always the case, and in some patients obesity becomes a problem, encouraged by lack of exercise and a high-carbohydrate food intake. This again must receive attention with an appropriate calorie-restricted diet, both on grounds of general health and because of the necessity of sparing diseased weight-bearing joints any additional burden.

Many patients are also concerned about their family and sexual life. There are probably inherited genetic factors which influence susceptibility to rheumatoid arthritis, but as pointed out in the previous chapter, these appear to be of limited overall importance and with certain exceptions there is not much in the way of hereditary predisposition. The man or woman with rheumatoid arthritis need therefore have little fear of passing the disease on to offspring. The effect of pregnancy itself is quite variable–some women notice no perceptible alteration in their symptoms, whereas others experience improvement during the later months of pregnancy, followed by a return of disease activity after delivery, an observation which is said to have stimulated the use of corticosteroid hormones in the treatment of the disorder. There is also some evidence to suggest that women with rheumatoid arthritis may be less fertile than others, though there are several possible causes for this. At all events, pregnancy in the long run appears to have no beneficial or deleterious effect, and should therefore be neither unduly encouraged or avoided for its own sake. On the other hand, a large family of young children presents a considerable physical and financial strain, so that family planning is important from this aspect. The contraceptive pill does not appear to alter the course of rheumatoid arthritis.

Patients are sometimes reluctant to seek advice about physical and emotional marital relationships and doctors to offer it, although most men and women are glad to discuss such problems given a suitable opportunity. Rather than engaging in direct conversation, some prefer the use of a booklet, such as the Arthritis and Rheumatism Council's *Marriage, sex and arthritis*, at least as a preliminary to the discussion of more individual difficulties. Arthritis like any other illness can certainly present physical and emotional obstacles to satisfying sexual intercourse. Lack of desire may be due to fatigue, often a prominent feature in rheumatoid arthritis, to pain or tenderness in joints, especially the hips, or perhaps occasionally to the effect of drugs in reducing libido. The marital partner should not interpret such reactions to coldness or frigidity in the ordinary sense of the term. Physical problems can usually be overcome by imaginative variation in traditional sexual techniques and postures—as one young lady patient remarked: 'There is more than one way of killing a cat'—but there is no doubt that the love, sympathy, and understanding which should form the basis of any marriage are especially requisite when one partner has rheumatoid arthritis.

It is inevitable that some people will try forms of treatment which are not usually employed by doctors, but which become fashionable from time to time—'fringe medicine'—such as new diets, acupuncture, and so on. Patients are often embarrassed to mention that they have done this, fearing the wrath that may fall upon them when it is learnt that they have strayed from the paths of medical orthodoxy. This should not be the case, however, and doctors are often interested to hear the results: knowing our own limitations, we can hardly blame the patient for trying something new. Purveyors of such remedies are usually ignorant, but they are by no means stupid and in their own interests they are unlikely to allow any great harm to be done. But some of these people are not exactly generous with their skills, and anger is an understandable reaction when one hears that a patient with rheumatoid arthritis has been persuaded to spend large sums of money, which she can often ill afford, on worthless bits of quackery.

Chronic disabling diseases where no cure is yet available lend themselves to all sorts of remedies and rheumatoid arthritis is no exception. There are hundreds of them, and my friend Dr. Frank Dudley Hart drew up an ABC of rheumatological remedies which is produced with his permission below.

The treatment of rheumatoid arthritis

Acupuncture; apple diet; auto-haemotherapy; angora wool
Bee venom; bangles, copper; baths, various
Chemotherapy; copper salts; crow's meat; cobalt
Doca and ascorbic acid; diet
Extractions of teeth and other septic foci; ECT
Fasting; fever; faith; fango
Gin; guaicum; gelatine; green-lipped mussel
Heat; honey; hope; hypnotism; hayseed
Insulin injections; iodine; inner cleanliness
Jaundice, induction of
K vitamin; kaolin compresses
Lourdes; love
Mud; magnetism; moxibustion; mistletoe
Nutmeg; nettles
Olive and other oils, oral and intra-articular
Placenta extracts; prayer; procaine; polyvinyl clothing
Quinine substitutes
Rhubarb; rest
Speransky's pump; sulphur; spa therapy; seaweed
Transfusions of blood, fresh or pregnant; tiger balm
Ultrasonics; underwear, anti-rheumatic; urea
Vitamins; vertebral manipulations; vaccines
Whale, standing inside; worms, earth-; water
Xmas snow
Yoghurt; yoga
Zam-buk; Zyloric (allopurinol)

There is not the space or necessity to discuss this formidable list. Copper bracelets have been worn to prevent or treat various types of arthritis for a good many years. It is uncertain how the custom arose: there is no reason to suppose that they can be of any use, but at least they are cheap, harmless, and to some extent decorative. Acupuncture—the insertion of fine needles into the skin—has been used for centuries but introduced into this country only relatively recently. It originated in China, where it is used today as a form of anaesthesia for major operations: theory cannot tell us why the procedure should be of any value. Controlled trials have been attempted in the U.S.A. with negative results.

Many patients are curious about people other than doctors who undertake the physical treatment of rheumatoid arthritis and allied disorders. I am referring here to osteopaths and chiropractors, who tend to practise independently, not to physiotherapists, occupational therapists, remedial gymnasts, pharmacists, and other invaluable members of the medical team, who work in collaboration with doctors. The place of physical treatment will be discussed in the next section: in so far as osteopaths and chiropractors may be skilled in such methods they serve a useful function, but in general they have nothing more to offer than the conventionally trained physiotherapist working in association with his or her medical colleagues. Little need be said of naturopaths, herbalists, and others, who have nothing to contribute beyond the psychological support and confidence which they may inspire (and which may be misplaced) and the hope, at least on their own part, that a natural remission in disease activity may take place during their ministrations.

Physical treatment

The term 'physical' here applies to methods of treatment which are basically mechanical, as opposed, for example, to those involving the use of drugs. The aim of physical treatment is the maintainence of function and the prevention of deformity; it is of the utmost importance in many patients with rheumatoid arthritis, especially in the more severely afflicted. Its principles are extremely simple but it is sometimes neglected by those who should know better. One of the problems with physical forms of treatment is the difficulty of carrying out controlled therapeutic trials, the importance of which has already been stressed. It is difficult to apply random allocation and 'double-blind' techniques to methods of treatment such as physiotherapy or surgical operation. Attempts have been made to carry out controlled trials to determine the value, for example, of bed-rest in rheumatoid arthritis, but the problems, as can be imagined, are considerable. Some years ago a group of hospital workers tried to assess in a controlled manner the effect of a particular form of heat treatment (in some patients, unbeknown to themselves or assessors, the switches were not turned on). Those receiving the treatment did no better than the others, and no beneficial effect could be attributed to the treatment.

Lacking evidence from controlled trials, the physician has to rely on his own experience or the fashion of the day. Both are fallible, but recommendation of the following forms of treatment is founded on pretty basic common sense: (a) bed rest; (b) active exercises; (c) splinting; (d) hydrotherapy; (e) others.

Bed rest

Despite the absence of controlled data, there is a generally accepted clinical impression that patients with active rheumatoid arthritis do better, at least in the short term, after a period—say three to four weeks—of bed rest and relative immobility. Pain and swelling in the joints tend to subside, as do general features of inflammation such as fever and an elevated sedimentation rate. It is also likely that the freedom from the pressure of everyday activities is beneficial.

Should a programme of bed rest be considered necessary, it should be carried out in a hospital rheumatology unit rather than at home. The opportunity can then be taken for careful observation and investigation of the disease, its complications, and the response to treatment, while instruction in exercises and splintage are also more easily undertaken. It cannot be too strongly emphasized that unsupervised rest in bed can be positively harmful and lead to permanent incapacity. Joints afflicted by rheumatoid arthritis tend not only to become restricted in their degrees of movement but to assume bad functional positions, particularly the knees, which easily become bent (flexion contracture), and the wrists, which similarly become fixed in a drooped position leading to a useless hand. The patient resting as shown in Plate 7(a) may be comfortable for a short time, but she will soon find herself deformed as shown in Plate 7(b), if indeed she is fortunate enough ever to get on her feet again. During periods of bed rest, therefore, constant attention must be paid to correct posture (see Plate 8). Even when our patient has resumed her normal life and activities, she should be encouraged to rest as much as possible, for example lying down for an hour after lunch.

Active exercises

The maintainance of function and the prevention of deformity are the principles every rheumatoid sufferer should always have in mind.

We have already seen the tendency of the knee and wrist to slip into flexion contracture, and these joints can be considered further as important examples of the general problem. The knee becomes bent (or flexed) by the action of the powerful hamstring muscles at the back of the thigh–you can feel their tendons behind each knee, one on each side, as you sit reading this book. Opposing the hamstrings, and thus preventing flexion contracture, are the muscles lying on the front of the thigh. This group of muscles is called the quadriceps, because it has four heads (or origins) all of which converge together to be inserted into the knee-cap and thence into the front of the shin-bone. The quadriceps muscles straighten (or extend) the knee, being used, for example, by a footballer when he kicks the ball.

There are various ways of educating and strengthening the quadriceps muscles–some of them quite fancy involving weights tied round the ankle and so on–but simple exercises are just as effective. There is nothing more simple or effective than the *static quadriceps exercises*, in which the patient is shown just how to contract and relax the quadriceps. This can easily be explained (see Plate 9). At first she is instructed to do the drill in the lying position on waking in the morning, during her mid-day rest, and on retiring at night–but she soon learns that the exercise can be carried out every few minutes, while standing at the sink, for example, or waiting for a bus. It has become instinctive, and she will never develop a flexion contracture of the knee. It is even easier to exercise the wrist. Anybody can learn to extend the wrist by exercising the appropriate muscles on the back of the forearm, and the action is soon performed habitually: never again will the wrist be allowed to droop over the lap or armchair. Once some one understands the frightful dangers of flexion contractures of the knee and wrist and how to avoid them a life-time of disability and deformity is avoided.

It has been said that active exercises should not be attempted while a joint is acutely inflamed. This is nonsense: it is at such times that exercise is most valuable to prevent as far as possible the muscle wasting that will otherwise take place. Such exercises have a bonus value if things go badly. If progressive deterioration takes place in a knee-joint, for example, and replacement surgery is considered, the surgeon will be delighted to have under his care a patient who is well-trained in quadriceps drill and whose chances of operative success will be so much the greater.

The wrist and knee joints have been taken as examples of basic principles. Similar considerations apply to other joints, but the emphasis is different: as we have seen, the loss of even a few degrees of full extension of the knee must be taken very seriously indeed, whereas loss of full extension of an elbow does not matter very much. Problems of individual joints are beyond the scope of this book and must be discussed by the patient with her own doctor and physiotherapist. It is worth making sure you have a few moments of the busy doctor's time in which he can explain and demonstrate these exercises. Sometimes the problem is more complicated: special joints may be involved, requiring special exercises, and some people are slower to learn the necessary techniques than others. In such situations the patient is referred to the physiotherapist, one of the most skilled members of the rheumatology team. Simplicity is still important: long lists of exercises tend to be self-defeating.

Splinting

Active exercise is all-important, but it is also necessary to prevent deformity during periods of repose, and this can be done by suitable splinting. Splinting can also protect the joint during active use of a limb. Splints for the wrist joint for use during rest and activity are shown in Plate 10.

Hydrotherapy

During or after periods of inflammation it may be difficult for a patient to maintain joint movement spontaneously. Many physiotherapeutic methods and gadgets are available to assist movement of a joint; in one method the therapist asks the patient to initiate a particular movement. The therapist helps the patient to continue the movement, and, after practice, unaided movement takes place. The use of a hydrotherapy pool is a most effective way of making movement easier; the buoyancy of the water relieves weight and its warmth tends to ease pain and muscle spasm (see Plate 11).

Other forms of physical treatment

Other methods are less important. Various forms of applied heat–hot packs or more elaborate appliances–may be a useful adjunct to exercise and movement. The rheumatoid sufferer should keep warm in cold weather, not scorning the use of knee warmers and other comforts. Slacks and trousers are a boon to many rheumatoid ladies.

Massage may be soothing but is otherwise of little use in rheumatoid arthritis. Passive movements and manipulation–where the limbs are moved by the therapist rather than by the patient–have a very limited part to play and may even be harmful.

Drugs

Many drugs are effective in helping to control the symptoms of rheumatoid arthritis but none can cure in the sense that an antibiotic, for example, will cure an infection caused by a sensitive micro-organism. There is a wide and unpredictable variation of response to drugs. Some of our anti-rheumatic drugs are potentially toxic, a fact which is generally and rightly appreciated but which must be kept in perspective. Numerous such drugs are now available, but the number to be prescribed for any one patient must obviously be kept to a minimum. Unfortunately our knowledge of their mode of action is rudimentary. The correct handling of drugs in rheumatoid arthritis is complicated and a detailed discussion of their pharmacology and toxicity is outside the scope of this book. It must suffice to outline the types of drugs which are in use and their place in treatment.

Non-steroidal anti-inflammatory drugs (NSAIDs)

Most patients with active rheumatoid arthritis require some form of medication to help them with their normal daily activities. Active exercise is often difficult in the face of joint and muscle stiffness, particularly the incapacitating morning stiffness with which the rheumatoid sufferer may awake but which can be considerably alleviated by NSAIDs. This is a large group of drugs, of many different types of chemical molecular structure, which combine the properties of pain relief (analgesia) with suppression of inflammation. The word 'non-steroidal' means that they do not include the corticosteroid hormones, to be discussed below. Although no active drug is completely without side-effects, the NSAIDs are relatively non-toxic and are widely prescribed. They are essentially symptomatic remedies, and it is intriguing to observe how some patients will benefit from one drug and some from another, so that individual patient preference is a matter of trial and error.

Table 4.1. NSAIDs available in Great Britain and (as noted) the United States*

Salicylates	Pyrazolones	Indolacetic acid derivatives
aspirin+ and its various preparations	phenylbutazone (Azolid: USA Butazolidin+ Butacote Sterazolidin: USA) oxyphenbutazone (Oxalid: USA Tandacote Tanderil+) azapropazone (Rheumox) feprazone (Methrazone)	indomethacin (Indocid Indocin: USA Artracin Imbrilon Tannex) sulindac (Clinoril+)
Propionic acid derivatives	**Arylacetic acid derivatives**	**Anthranilic acid derivatives**
ibuprofen (Brufen, Ebufac, Motrin: USA) fenbufen (Lederfen) flurbiprofen (Froben) fenoprofen (Fenopron, Progesic, Nalfon: USA) ketoprofen (Orudis, Alrheumat) naproxen (Naprosyn+, Synflex) benoxaprofen (Opren)	diclofenac (Voltarol) fenclofenac (Flenac) tolmetin (Tolectin+)	mefenamic acid (Ponstan Ponstel: USA) also piroxicam (Feldene)

*Examples of proprietary (trade) names are given in brackets.
+Available in the United States under the same name.

Aspirin (acetyl salicylic acid) has by far the longest lineage—nearly 100 years of undiminished usefulness and popularity, 4000 million tablets being swallowed every year in Great Britain. Many patients with rheumatoid arthritis find that it provides adequate relief from their pain and stiffness, if taken in adequate dosage, and it has been called the 'sheet anchor' of treatment. Some, however, find difficulty in tolerating high doses for prolonged periods, even in such formulations as soluble aspirin or coated tablets, so that one of the other NSAIDs is then preferable. Serious toxicity from aspirin is extremely rare. Unlike the analgesic compound phenacetin (no longer prescribed) it does not, alone and in therapeutic dosage, cause kidney damage; it does cause a low-grade gastritis and bleeding from the stomach, but this is usually trivial and of no practical importance.

Patients often ask if such drugs are merely 'pain-killers'. They are rather more important than that, since they can be shown to suppress inflammation in clinical and experimental studies, as opposed to pure analgesic preparations such as paracetamol (Panadol) and dextropropoxyphene (contained in Distalgesic). On the other hand, it is unlikely that in themselves they influence the long term course of the disease to any significant degree.

Drugs with a more specific action

While the majority of patients with rheumatoid arthritis will do well on one or other of the NSAIDs, a proportion will continue to show evidence of continued disease activity with progressive joint damage, indicated by the appearance and development of erosions as shown on X-rays. Such patients will generally require one of a group of drugs which appear to suppress the activity of rheumatoid arthritis, and perhaps slow down its rate of evolution, on a long-term basis. These drugs have no obvious immediate effect, and any response takes several weeks to become apparent.

Gold (Myocrisin) was introduced into the treatment of rheumatoid arthritis 50 years ago. Given by intramuscular injection, usually at weekly intervals, gold is effective in a proportion of patients after a delay of two to three months and it can be continued in low dosage over a period of years. In the absence of careful supervision, however, gold can be dangerously toxic. A skin rash or ulceration of the mouth is the most common side-effect; damage to the kidneys is not uncommon but rarely severe. The most serious side-effect is suppression of production of the cells in the bone marrow–platelets, white cells, and red cells. Complete suppression can lead to aplastic anaemia, which is sometimes fatal. It is therefore necessary for the physician to test the urine and examine the blood at frequent intervals; if due care is taken gold is a useful drug and serious toxic complications can nearly always be avoided.

More recently a drug called penicillamine (Distamine, Depamine)—not to be confused with the antibiotic penicillin, although there is some chemical similarity between the two drugs—has come to be used in the treatment of rheumatoid arthritis. It is taken in tablet form but is otherwise remarkably similar to gold both in its therapeutic efficacy and in the nature of its more serious side-effects. There is therefore little to choose between the two. The use of penicillamine, like gold, must be scrupulously monitored.

The introduction of many drugs of this sort has been due in the first place to rather fortuitous reasoning: for example, gold salts were used because it was thought that they were effective in the treatment of tuberculosis (which they are not) and that rheumatoid arthritis was a form of tuberculosis (which it is not). Some years ago it was observed that some anti-malarial drugs, such as chloroquine or hydroxychloroquine (Plaquenil), had a similar delayed beneficial effect, albeit not usually a very powerful one, and controlled trials appear to have confirmed this. The anti-malarials are free of the potentially lethal side-effects which can be caused by gold and penicillamine, but they can cause serious damage to the eyes. Again, however, with careful dosage and ophthalmic supervision they are generally safe enough.

Corticosteroids

'Gentlemen, this is no humbug', growled Walter Bauer, the sceptical elder statesman of American rheumatology, when the effect of cortisone, one of the hormones of the adrenal gland, was demonstrated to him in 1949. Certainly anything as dramatic can seldom have been seen in the history of medicine, as stiff, immobile rheumatoid cripples walked and jumped, free of pain. The honeymoon period was soon over, as it became realized that the dosage of cortisone required to suppress the disease—and it did no more than that—produced also an alarming concatenation of toxic effects, ranging from the unsightly and hairy 'moon-face' to perforating and bleeding gastric ulceration.

Further, the drug did nothing to heal rheumatoid erosions of cartilage and bone, nor did it appear to have any effect on the long-term course of the disease. Physicians recoiled from this two-edged weapon.

Opinions remain divided, but 30 years' experience has taught us a great deal about these hormones and their place in the treatment of rheumatoid arthritis and other inflammatory disorders of connective tissue. The drug usually employed is prednisone (or prednisolone, pharmacologically identical) which has a similar action to cortisone, to which it is structurally related. We have learnt to use prednisone in low dosage, when it is relatively harmless, in patients in whom active disease is not controlled by NSAIDs. It is sometimes prescribed in combination for a time with gold or penicillamine; and although it remains true that the physician starting a patient on 'steroids' must reckon with the necessity of life-long treatment, nevertheless it is usually possible to confine the dosage to acceptable levels and often gradually to withdraw the drug completely after a period of disease activity. A controlled, knowledgeable, and dynamic approach to their use is essential. The chronic arthritic on 10 milligrams of prednisolone daily year in, year out is almost certainly not benefiting from the imaginative flexibility which is necessary in the prescribing of these drugs.

Other drugs

Compounds used in the treatment of cancer—for example cyclophosphamide and azathioprine—have been tested in rheumatoid arthritis and have been considered to exert a slight but definite anti-rheumatic effect, though whether this is due to an influence upon immunological activity, cellular proliferation, or simply inflammation is uncertain. They are toxic drugs with numerous side-effects, including marrow suppression, and they are not used routinely. Levamisole is a drug which has been used in parasitic infections for a number of years: it too influences the immune response and preliminary studies indicate that it has a therapeutic and toxic activity comparable to gold and penicillamine. Its use may still be regarded as experimental.

At a less esoteric level, the usefulness of pure analgesics has already been mentioned. Sedatives and anti-depressant drugs also have a beneficial effect when prescribed judiciously, but insomnia and depression are of course usually secondary to the disease itself, which must be the main target of therapy. Vitamins and iron are indicated when there is evidence of deficiency but in themselves have no anti-rheumatic effect.

Local injection of drugs

Occasionally a single joint remains troublesome even when the disease has become quiescent elsewhere. This applies particularly to the knee joint where the extensive area of synovial membrane predisposes to recurrent, painful effusion. This often responds well to the removal of the fluid with syringe and needle together with injection of a steroid preparation: the patient need have no worry about the side-effects which can occur when steroids are administered systemically. Another procedure, the use of which is confined to a few specialized centres, consists of treating active synovitis with a radioactive substance such as radioactive yttrium.

Surgery

The increasing application of orthopaedic surgery to the management of rheumatoid arthritis during the past 20 years has been a major therapeutic advance. Surgeons formerly knew little of the disease and were reluctant to operate on actively inflamed joints, but they are now very knowledgeable about the pathology of rheumatoid arthritis and the role which they themselves have to play. As their traditional source of clinical material from tuberculosis and poliomyelitis has dwindled and as operative techniques, particularly the development of joint replacement by artificial joints (prostheses), have improved, so rheumatoid arthritis and other forms of arthritis have come to occupy a much larger proportion of the orthopaedic work-load.

For the best results, the selection of suitable cases is vital, and the orthopaedic surgeon relies here upon careful assessment in collaboration with the rheumatologist, who must also remain responsible for the continuation of medical care during the operative period, which is but an episode in the patient's long-term management. The state of the patient's general health and the presence and severity of disease in other joints apart from that upon which the operation is being considered must be taken into account before surgery takes place. Although heroic programmes involving several joints are now successfully undertaken–all rheumatologists for example, have under their care a handful of cases in which both hips and both knees have been replaced–the ideal subject is one in whom the general health is good and severe damage is limited to one or two joints.

The aims of surgical treatment are threefold: improvement in function, relief of pain, and improvement in appearance. The last is a rare indication for surgery, which is hardly ever carried out for cosmetic reasons alone. There are three major types of operation used on the joints of patients with rheumatoid arthritis.

Synovectomy

In this procedure the surgeon removes as much of the inflamed synovial membrane as possible, with the object of reducing the amount of pain and swelling. The operation is usually highly successful, for example, in dealing with recurrent effusions in a knee joint which has not responded satisfactorily to intra-articular steroid or yttrium. Hopes that the operation, by removing diseased tissue, may retard the eventual rate of joint damage remain unsubstantiated. It is general experience that synovectomy is now performed less frequently than was the case a few years ago: perhaps this is a testimony to the increasing effectiveness of medical treatment with drugs such as gold and penicillamine.

Arthroplasty

This term applies to any procedure which reconstitutes a joint, either by simple excision of damaged joint surfaces or by the more sophisticated techniques of joint replacement. Replacement arthroplasty, using metal and plastic prostheses, is well established in hip surgery (see Plate 12) and has more recently become so in the knee. Prosthetic replacements of the shoulder, elbow, and ankle are also being developed and are certainly greatly needed. Artificial joints for the fingers have been used for many years, but the numerous varieties of finger joint prothesis currently available confirm that none is really satisfactory. On the other hand, simple excision arthroplasty of the toe joints is one of the most effective and rewarding operations in rheumatology. Joint replacement is normally indicated when a joint has become extensively damaged by the disease process with resulting severe pain and disability. Surgical techniques vary to a considerable extent depending on the type of joint involved. In the example shown in Plate 13 the surgeon has removed the diseased head of the femur (thigh bone) replacing it with a metal ball which is secured downwards into the shaft of the bone. A plastic socket, into which the ball fits, has been inserted into the pelvic part of the joint. In properly selected patients the results of surgery are gratifying with relief of pain and rapid mobilisation after operation. Complications, such as loosening of the prosthesis or secondary infection, though serious when they occur, are rare.

This question of selection is all-important. Whereas in osteoarthrosis of the hip (Chapter 6, p. 64) the surgeon is usually dealing with a single joint in an otherwise healthy person, the rheumatoid patient presents a problem of multiple joint involvement against a background of general illness, limiting the scope of possible surgical intervention.

Arthrodesis

Fixation of a joint in a good functional position, derived either from nature or the surgeon's art is by no means an unsatisfactory end-result. Surgical fixation, or arthrodesis, is less frequently performed nowadays because of the increasing availability of prosthetic replacements. Nevertheless, arthrodesis effectively removes pain and corrects instability; it is still of great value in the thumb, wrist, elbow, and ankle joints.

Other orthopaedic and plastic operations performed in rheumatoid arthritis include the repair of tendons damaged by the disease (sometimes a matter of considerable urgency), complex operations to stabilize vertebrae in the neck, and thus prevent progressive pressure on the spinal cord, and removal of rheumatoid nodules. There is also an operation called osteotomy, in which the bone is divided outside the joint capsule with the object of altering the mechanics of weight transmission and the pattern of blood flow: this operation is of questionable value.

Rehabilitation

The term 'rehabilitation' may be taken to signify the whole process of restoring a disabled person to a condition in which he is able, as far as possible, to resume a normal life; it embraces all the physical, social, and organizational aspects of aftercare. It is naturally an important part of the management of any chronic disorder, but, as pointed out in Chapter 1, the specific association of 'Rheumatology and Rehabilitation', a designation of a medical speciality still used by the Department of Health and Social Security in England, represents an outmoded concept. Nevertheless, organized integration of medical, social, educational, and industrial requirements of severely handicapped people in regional rehabilitation units has much to commend it.

The importance of adequate discussion with patient and family has already been emphasized, and the various types of physical treatment outlined. The changing nature of the disease, with altering physical and psychological capability, means that repeated functional *assessment* is necessary, so that the aims of treatment can remain clearly defined. Medical staff, physiotherapists, occupational therapists, and medical social workers all have a part to play; practical assessment in the patient's home should not be omitted.

Re-settlement in work depends on many factors such as the severity of the disease, nature of the work, and educational background. Heavy manual work may have to be changed. Sometimes travel to and from work is the limiting factor rather than the job itself. The best results are often obtained by informal arrangements depending on the initiative of the patient, his friends, relatives, employer, and doctor, but the services of disablement resettlement officers, industrial rehabilitation units, and government training centres are sometimes necessary. Nor should the importance of maintaining leisure interests and hobbies be forgotten.

Most patients with rheumatoid arthritis continue to lead relatively normal lives, but they may have to overcome some limitation of function. Numerous types of 'aids to daily living' are available from hospitals, local authorities, and voluntary bodies (Plate 13). These include: bath and toilet aids (for example bath seats, handles, raised W. C. seats), dressing aids (for example stocking aids, adapted clothing, and shoes), walking aids (for example sticks and frames), eating aids (for example special eating utensils), and household aids (for example pick-up sticks, bookrests). More elaborate adaptation may be required in the design of the home, fittings, and furniture, such as: high backed chairs and footstools, sometimes with 'ejection seats', adapted kitchen equipment (long-handled taps, special working surfaces), lever-handled windows, tilting beds, and hoists. For bed-bound patients, remote-control devices are available whereby switches will operate lights, television, the opening of front doors and so on. An example of such a system is POSSUM (Patient Operated Selector Mechanism). Aids to mobility include the provision of many different types of self-propelling or electrically powered wheelchairs, invalid vehicles, and mobility allowances. Generous provision is made for these by the National Health Service. Responsibility for assessment and provision of facilities lies with each Regional Medical Officer and his nominated assessors.

I have given only a brief outline of rehabilitation services in this book. More detailed information can be obtained from publications such as the following: *Living with a handicap* by P. Nichols (1974). Priory Press, London. The series 'Equipment for the Disabled' (published by the Oxford Regional Health Authority: orders to 2 Foredown Drive, Portslade, Sussex BN4 2BB). *Aids for handicapped people* (1975). British Red Cross Society. Advice may also be obtained from the agencies listed at the end of this book.

5

Ankylosing spondylitis and other related forms of arthritis

Rheumatoid arthritis is only one of many different types of chronic inflammatory arthritis, and in this chapter we shall consider a few of the other varieties. Some of these have been confused in the past with rheumatoid arthritis. For example, ankylosing spondylitis (a term derived from the Greek *ankylos* meaning stiffening of a joint and *spondylos* meaning a vertebra) was for a time called 'rheumatoid spondylitis' under the mistaken impression that it was a variant of rheumatoid arthritis involving predominantly the vertebral column; I can remember as a medical student listening to long discussions about whether or not rheumatoid arthritis was more common in people who had the skin disease psoriasis, held without any clear concept of psoriatic arthritis as a separate disease entity. Subsequently, however, it was realized that rheumatoid factor, present in the serum of most patients with rheumatoid arthritis (Chapter 3, page 22), was absent from patients with these other conditions, which therefore came to be called 'seronegative'. Further distinctions were appreciated, and the high frequency of the histocompatability antigen HLA B27, a factor found in the blood in cases of ankylosing spondylitis, as will shortly be described, is not a feature of rheumatoid arthritis.

Ankylosing spondylitis

This is an inflammatory disease of the spine affecting predominantly young men. It is probably less common than rheumatoid arthritis, and epidemiological studies indicate a prevalence of about 0·1 per cent in the general population. It shows a very strong tendency to run in families.

Inflammation, the underlying cause of which is unknown, commences as microscopic accumulation of cells at sites where ligaments leave bone, especially where the fibres of the annulus fibrosus of the intervertebral disc (Chapter 2, page 18) are attached to the edges of vertebrae. The bone responds to this by growing out along the edges of the annulus, the outer fibres of which become ossified. In fully developed forms of the disease, therefore, the vertebrae become fused; the back loses its flexibility and becomes rigid ('poker back' or 'bamboo spine'–Plate 14). Other pathological changes include inflammation and fusion of the sacro-iliac joints at the base of the spine (*sacro-iliitis*) and erosive arthritis in the peripheral joints of the body very similar to rheumatoid arthritis. As with rheumatoid arthritis there are non-articular features: rheumatoid nodules and vasculitis are not found, but episodes of inflammation of the eye (iritis) occur in about one-fifth of patients and may be the first symptom of the disease. Much less common are cardiovascular complications, which include inflammatory changes in the aorta and aortic valve of the heart. Loosening (subluxation) of the attachments between the upper two vertebrae, the atlas and the axis, can occasionally lead to pressure upon the spinal cord with consequent neurological damage.

Symptoms

Symptoms of the disease usually start rather insidiously with aching and stiffness in the lower back, worse on rising in the morning and improved by mild exercise. At first the pain occurs in bouts lasting a few days, later becoming more continuous; the pattern is quite variable and often there is very little pain at all. In some patients the pain closely resembles that of sciatica due to a lumbar disc injury (Chapter 11). Pain is sometimes localized to the chest and in some patients, particularly children, the first symptom may be in a peripheral joint such as the knee or ankle. The hips and shoulders are also involved quite frequently.

Physical examination in the early stages of the disease may reveal no abnormality, or perhaps just a little restriction of movement in the lumbar vertebrae. Later, the normal curvature of the lumbar spine is lost and its mobility becomes clearly limited, as does the ability to expand the chest fully on taking a deep breath. There is a tendency to develop a characteristic posture, especially in untreated cases: the head and neck are held forwards, the upper back is rounded, and the chest flattened.

The pathological changes in the vertebral column, from sacro-iliitis to advanced lesions such as the 'bamboo spine' can easily be seen in X-rays. X-rays of the sacro-iliac joints are especially useful because detection of sacro-iliitis by clinical examination is unreliable. As with other inflammatory diseases, the erythrocyte sedimentation rate is elevated, but tests for rheumatoid factor are negative.

Cause

As with so many of the rheumatic diseases, we understand little of the causation of ankylosing spondylitis, but recent years have seen some advances in knowledge. The strong familial aggregation of ankylosing spondylitis has been appreciated for many years, and the importance of genetic factors has been emphasized by the realization that there is a close link between the disease and the presence of the histo-compatability antigen HLA B27. It is generally known that we all belong to one of a number of blood groups according to the presence of blood group antigens situated on red cells: transfusion with in-compatible blood may lead to an adverse 'transfusion reaction'. In a comparable way there is another system of antigens situated on the surfaces of lymphocytes and other cells. They are responsible for rejection by the host of a graft from another animal of the same species. Identification of these histocompatability antigens is of course an important investigation in the field of transplantation surgery, such as kidney or heart transplantation. The cells of any individual possess four varieties of histocompatability (or HLA, Human Leucocyte Antigen) antigens, two being derived from each parent. The genes responsible for the production of such antigens, which influence the compatability of tissues and other types of intercellular reactions, are situated on a small segment of a particular (the sixth) chromosome, the region being known as the major histocompatability complex (MHC).

There are numerous examples in medicine of associations between an individual disease and the presence of particular HLA antigens (of which there are a very large number), but none is more striking than that which exists between ankylosing spondylitis and HLA B27. Present in only 7 per cent of the normal population, HLA B27 is

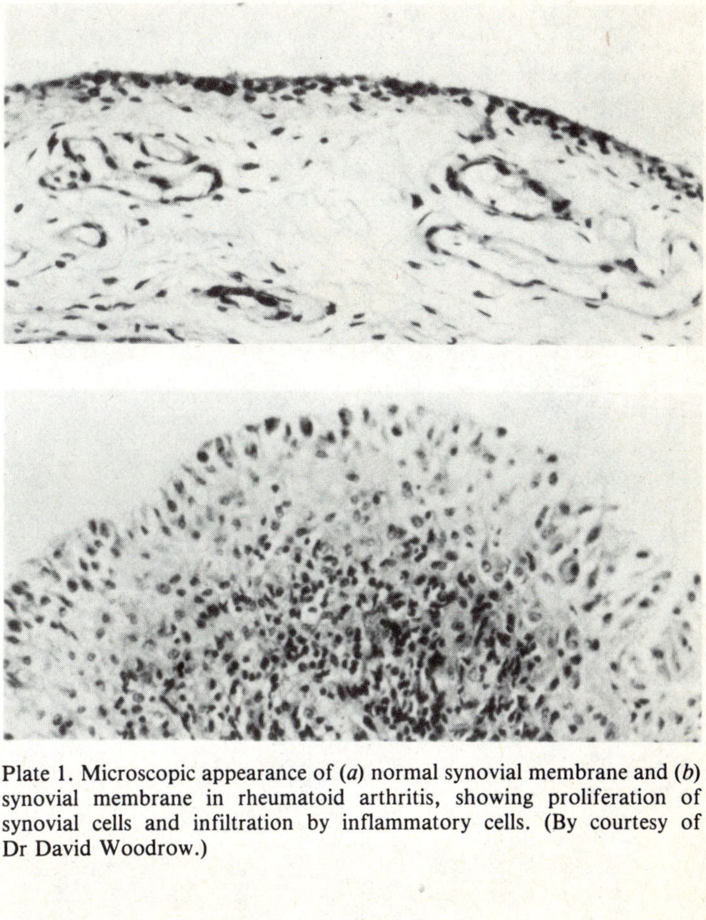

(a)

(b)

Plate 1. Microscopic appearance of (*a*) normal synovial membrane and (*b*) synovial membrane in rheumatoid arthritis, showing proliferation of synovial cells and infiltration by inflammatory cells. (By courtesy of Dr David Woodrow.)

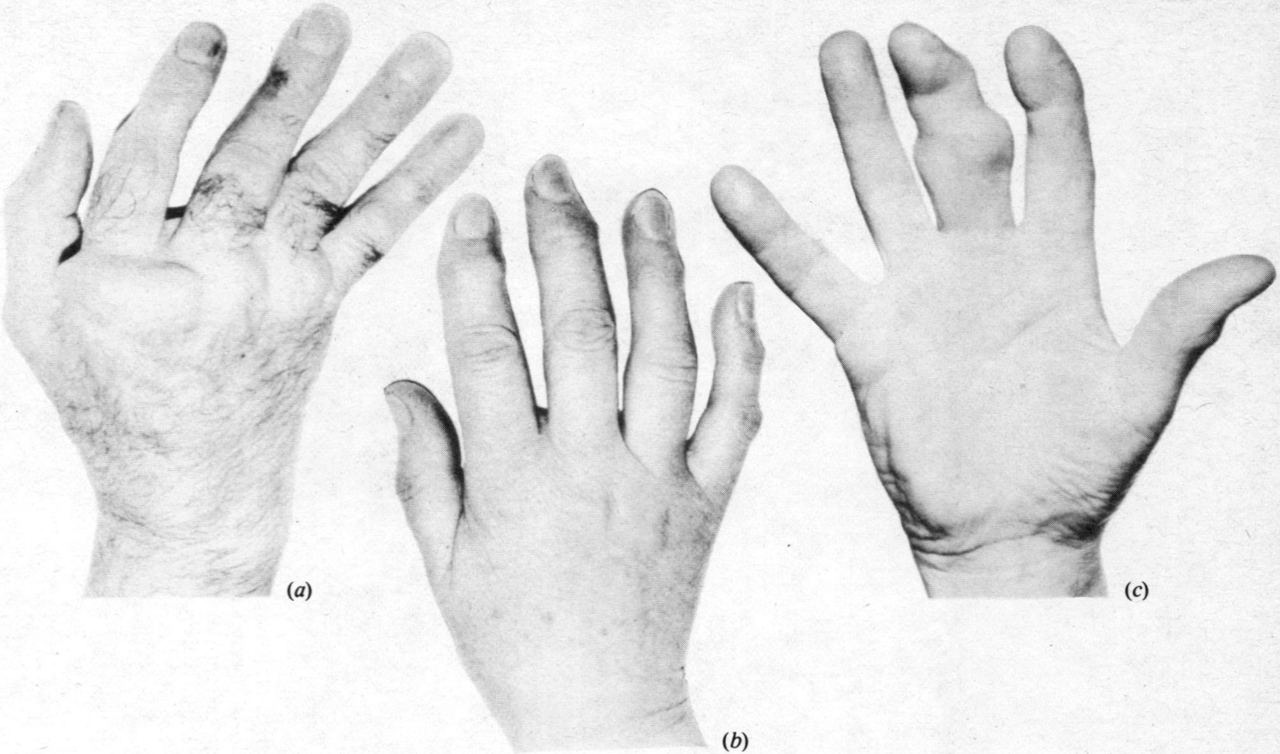

Plate 2. Appearance of the hand in (*a*) rheumatoid arthritis, (*b*) osteoarthrosis, and (*c*) gout.

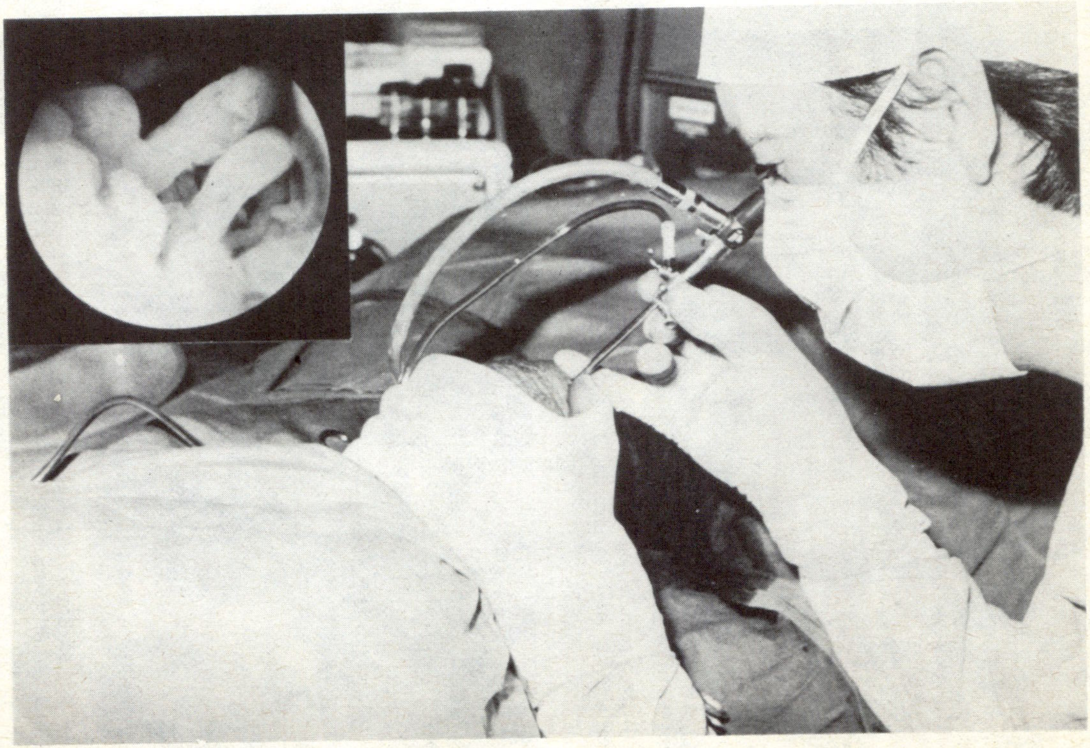

Plate 3. Direct visualization of the interior of the knee joint using an arthroscope. (Inset top left: the appearance through the arthroscope of the rheumatoid synovial membrane with its villi.)

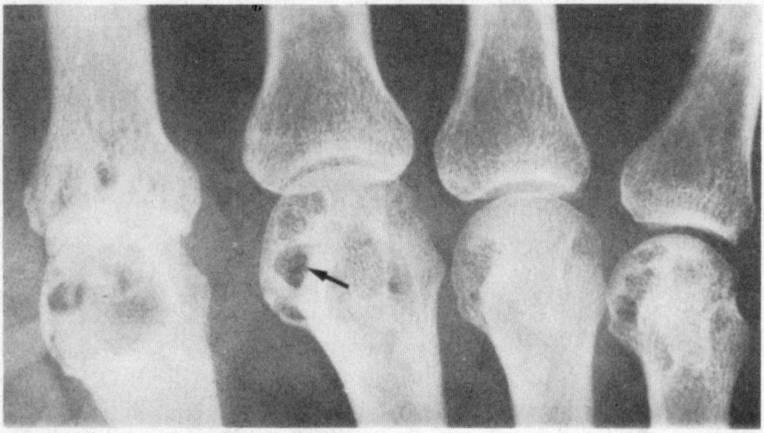

Plate 4. Deep punched-out erosions in the hand of a patient with rheumatoid arthritis who had never taken a day off his work as a railway porter.

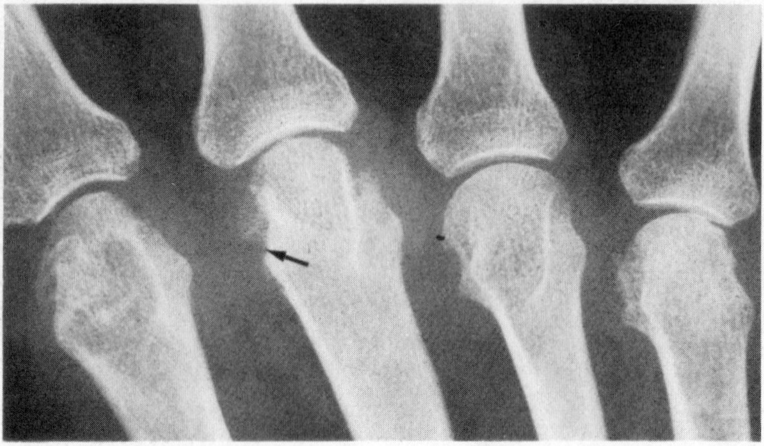

Plate 5. Shallow superficial erosions in the hand of a young woman with rheumatoid arthritis: she made little effort to maintain her normal level of physical activity.

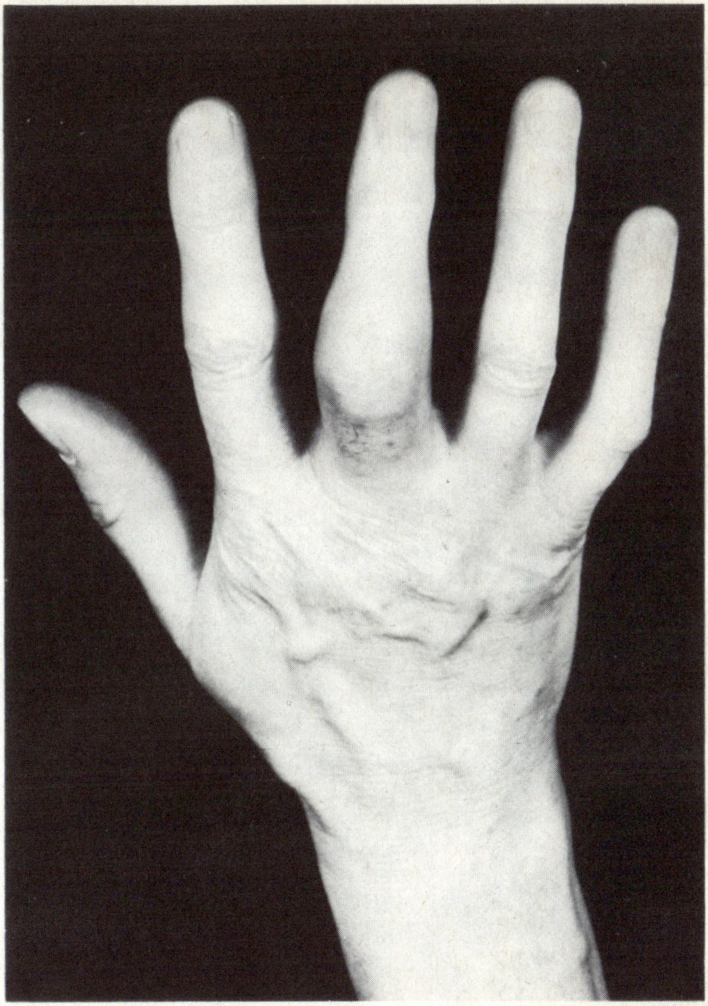

Plate 6. Predominant involvement of a finger joint in a patient with early generalized rheumatoid arthritis: the joint had been injured just before he developed signs of the disease.

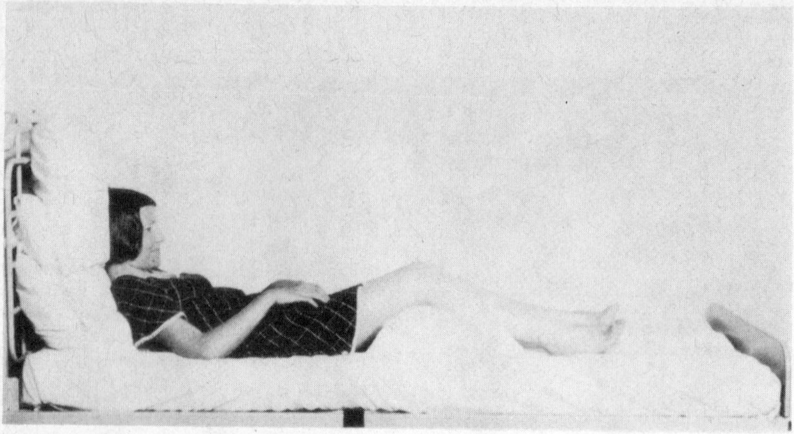

(*a*)

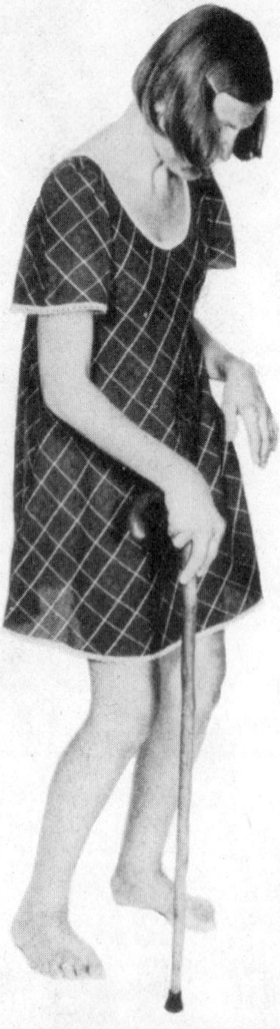

(*b*)

Plate 7. (*a*) Bed rest with harmful posture: flexion of neck, elbows, wrists, hips, and knees. (*b*) Resultant difficulty in walking.

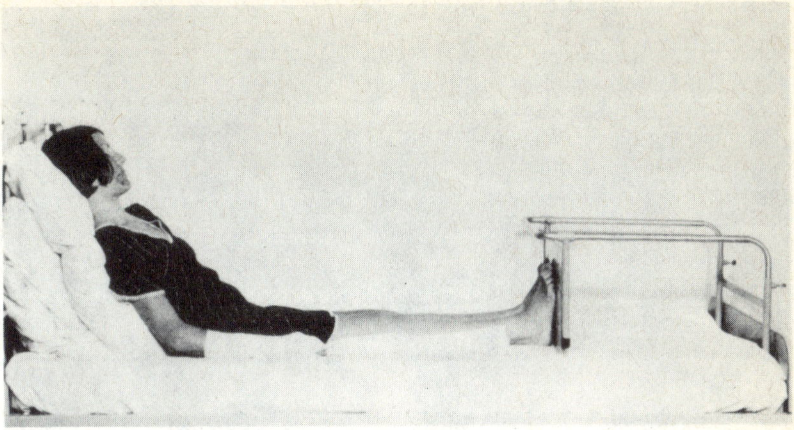

(*a*)

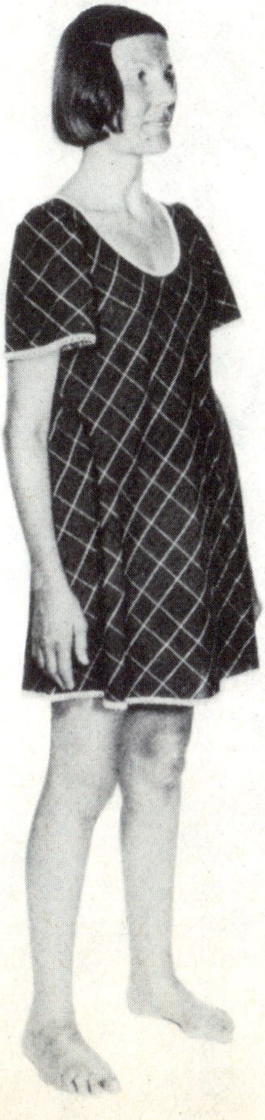

(*b*)

Plate 8. (*a*) and (*b*) Better functional position.

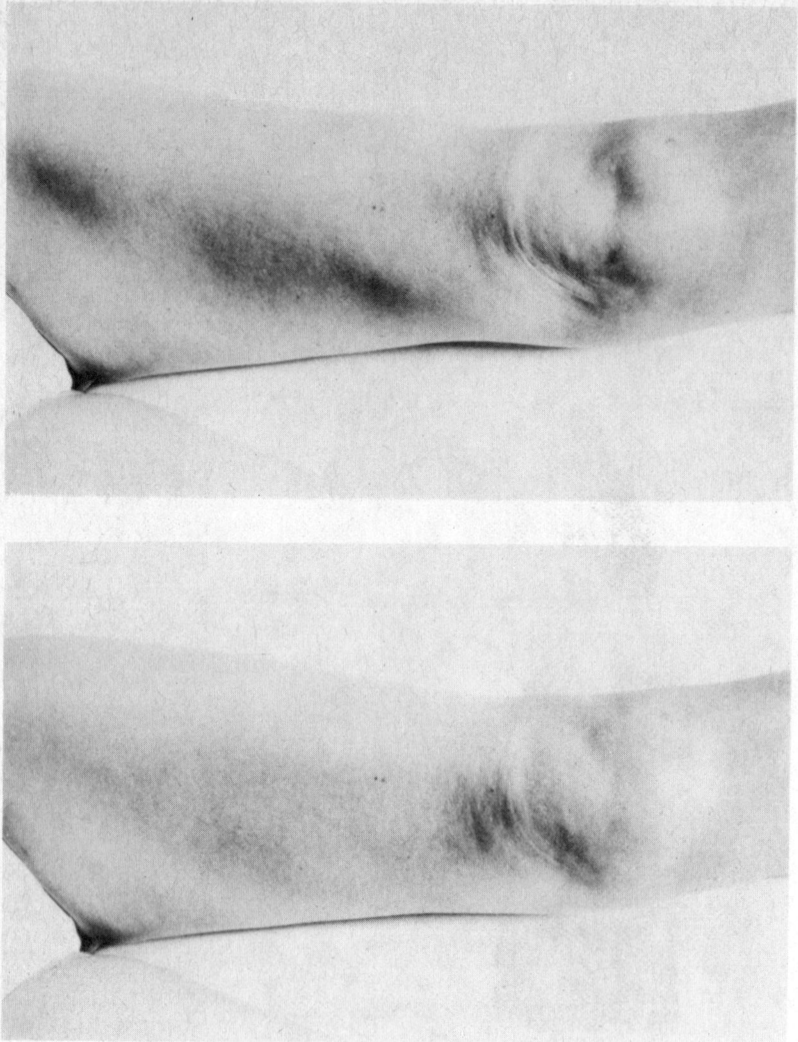

(*a*)

(*b*)

Plate 9. Static quadriceps exercise: (*a*) contraction; (*b*) relaxation.

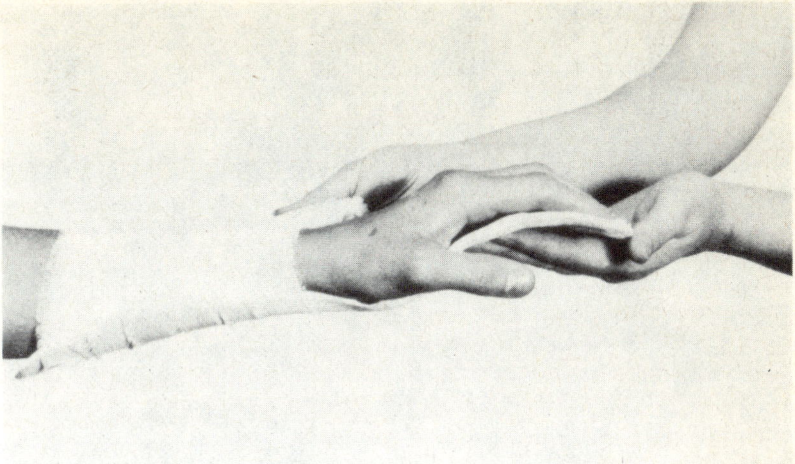

(*a*)

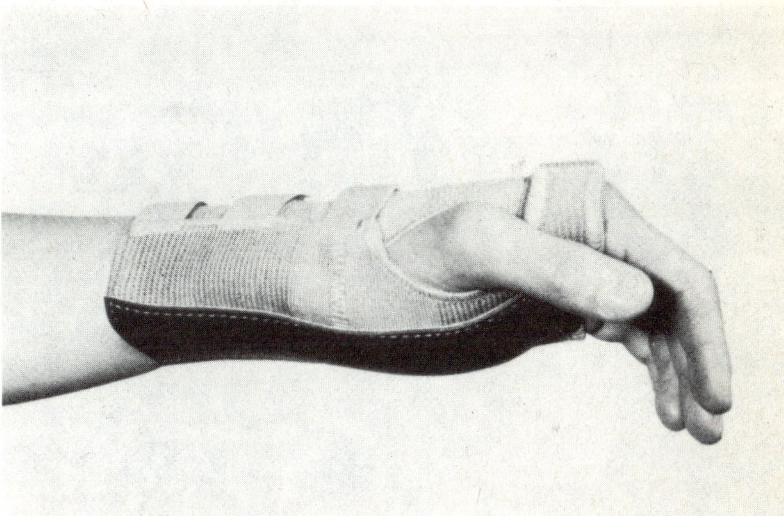

(*b*)

Plate 10. Splints for the wrist joint for use during (*a*) rest and (*b*) physical activity (Futura splint).

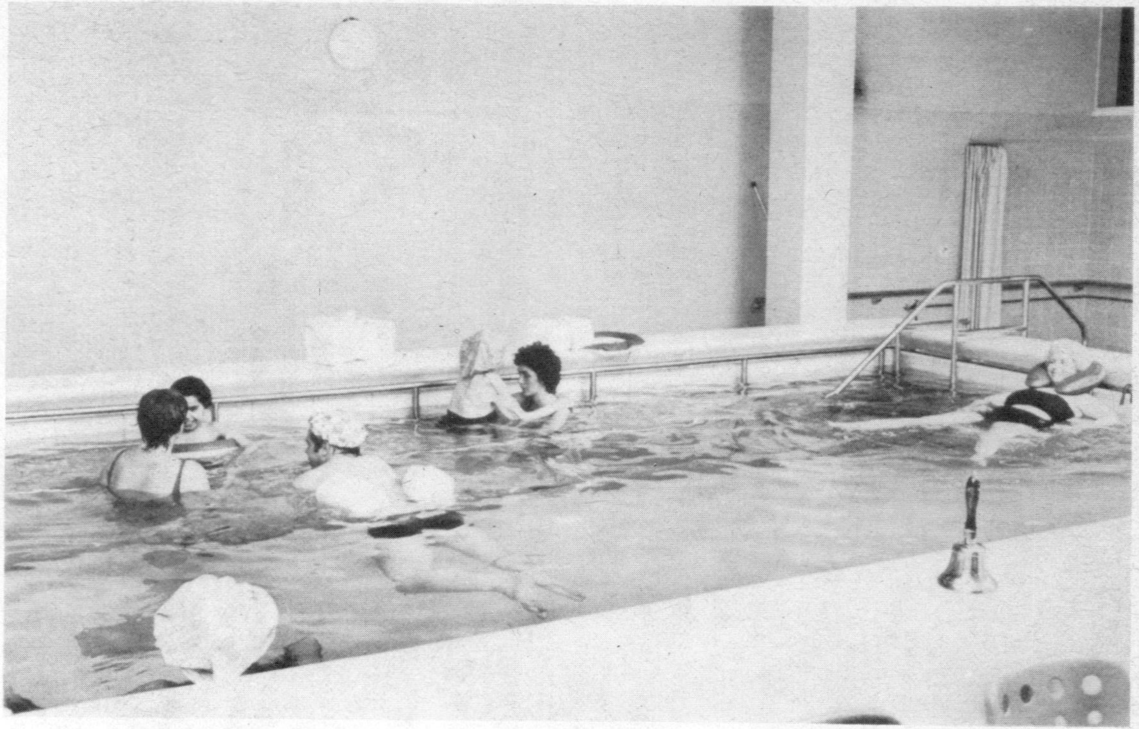

Plate 11. Hydrotherapy pool, Charing Cross Hospital.

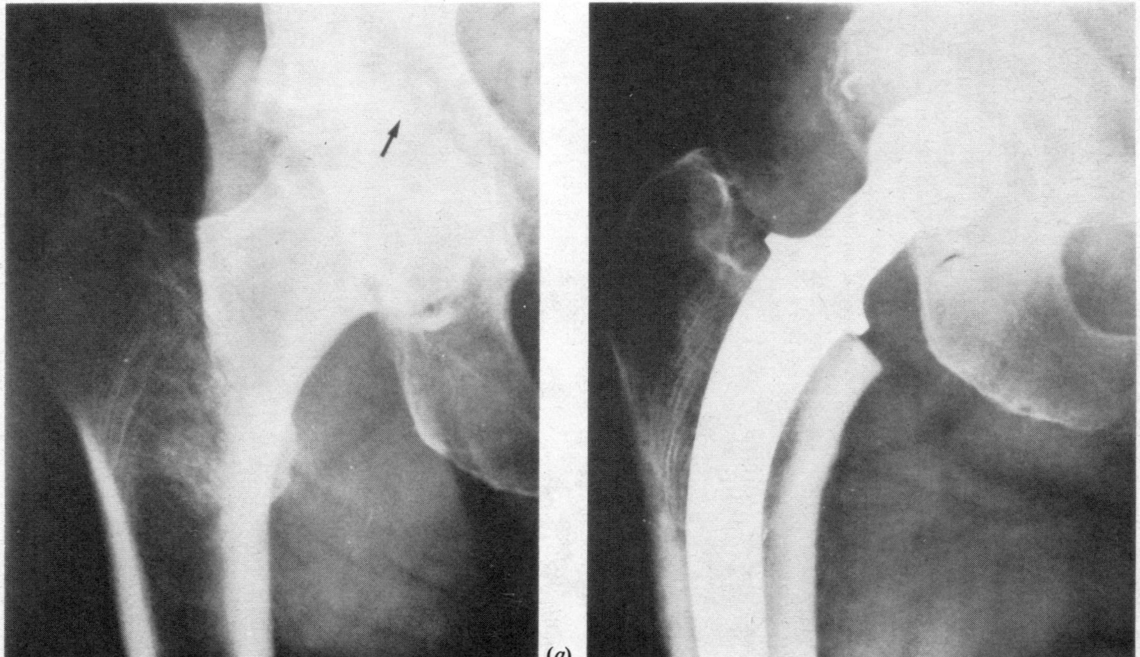

(*a*) (*b*)

Plate 12. X-ray of rheumatoid hip joint (*a*) before and (*b*) after total hip replacement. In (*a*) the narrowed joint space, due to destruction of articular cartilage, is arrowed.

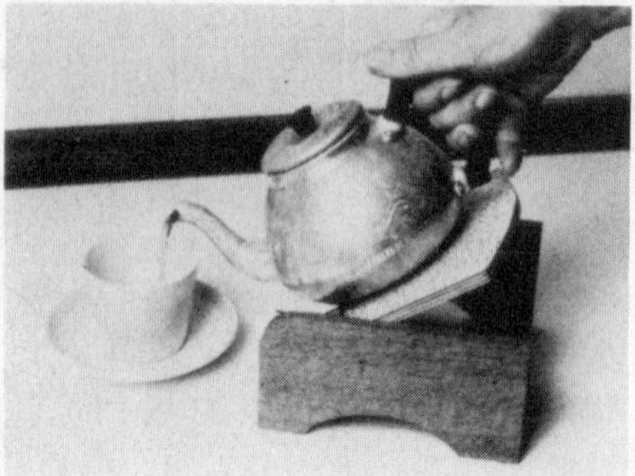

(*a*)

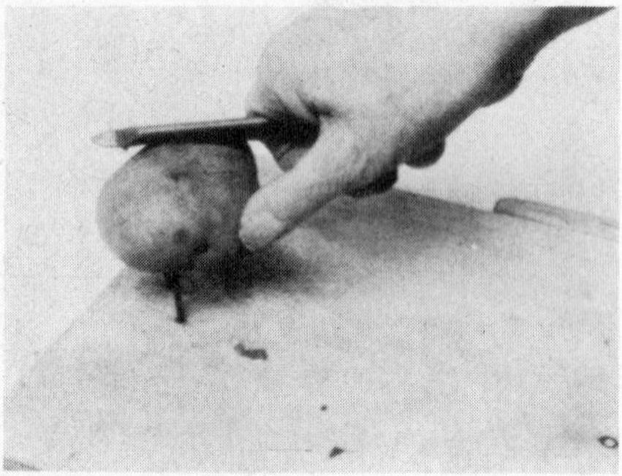

(*b*)

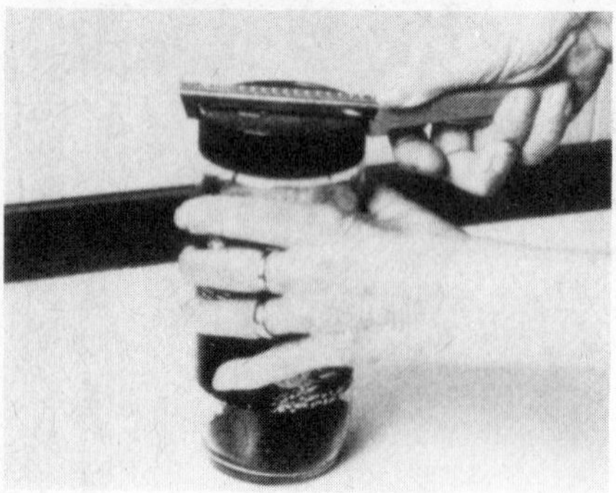

(*c*)

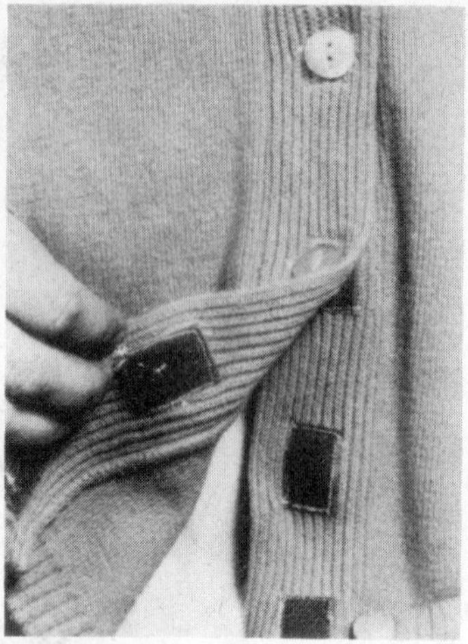

(*d*)

Plate 13. Examples of 'aids to daily living'. (*a*) Tea-pot support; (*b*) board with spikes for peeling potatos; (*c*) gadget for unscrewing jar tops; (*d*) Velcro adhesive to replace buttons.

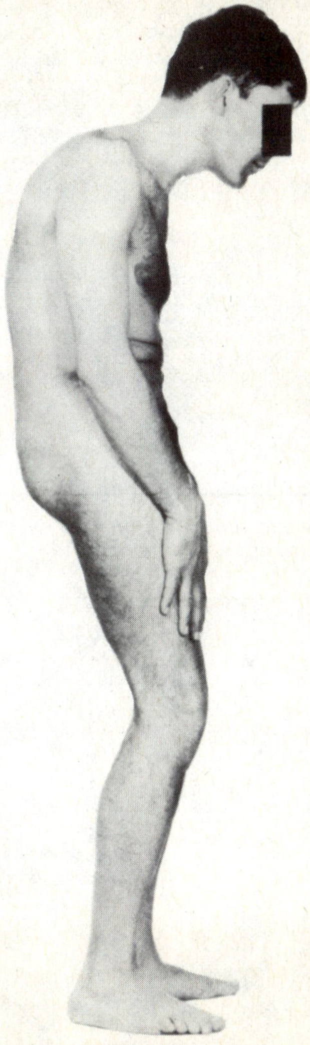

Plate 14. Ankylosing spondylitis.

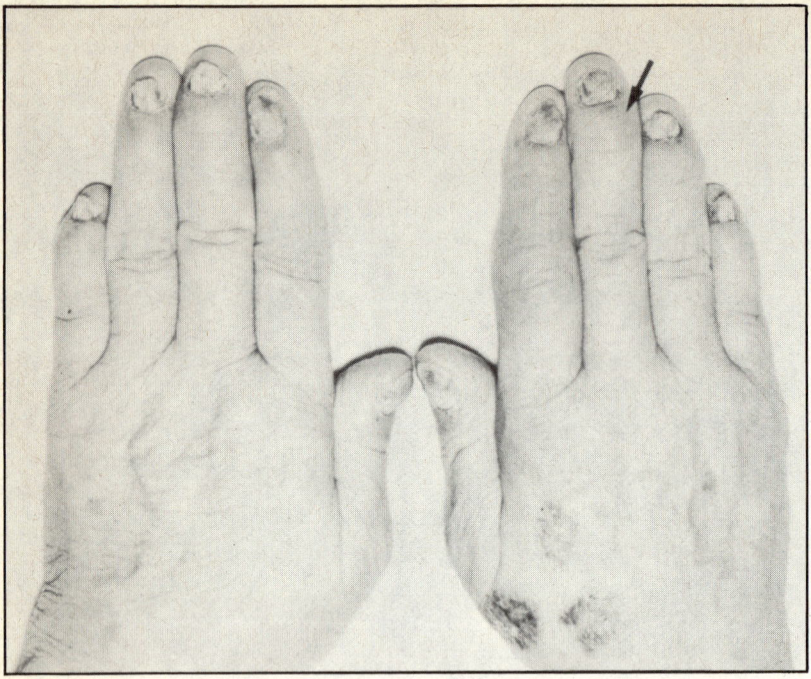

Plate 15. Hands of a patient with psoriatic arthritis. Psoriasis is seen involving the skin and finger-nails. The swelling of the joints is arrowed.

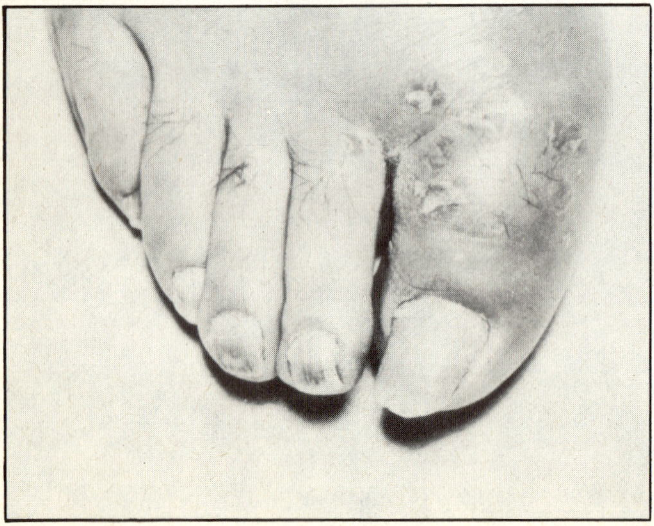

Plate 16. Acute gouty arthritis in a great toe.

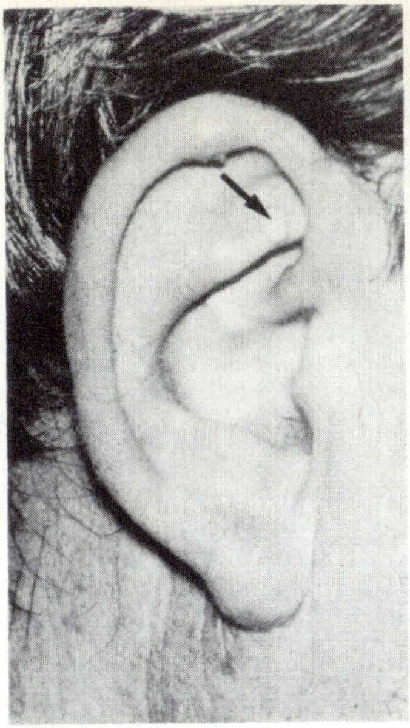

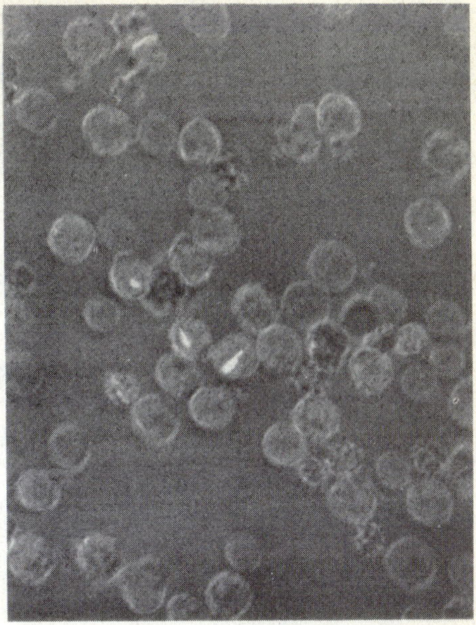

Plate 17. Gouty tophus on an ear lobe.

Plate 18. Crystals of sodium urate lying within inflammatory cells as seen by microscopy of a sample of joint fluid from a patient with gout.

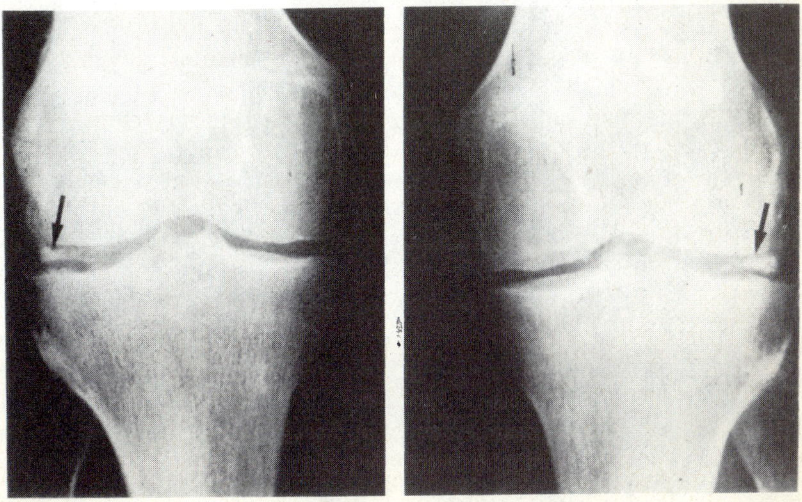

Plate 19. X-ray of the knees from a patient with chondrocalcinosis showing calcification within the menisci (arrowed).

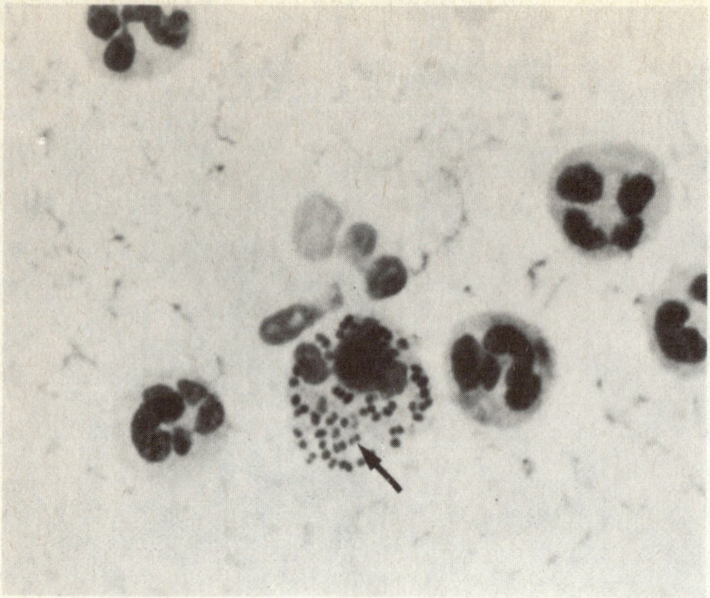

Plate 20. Joint fluid from a case of gonococcal infective arthritis: gonococci are seen lying within inflammatory cells.

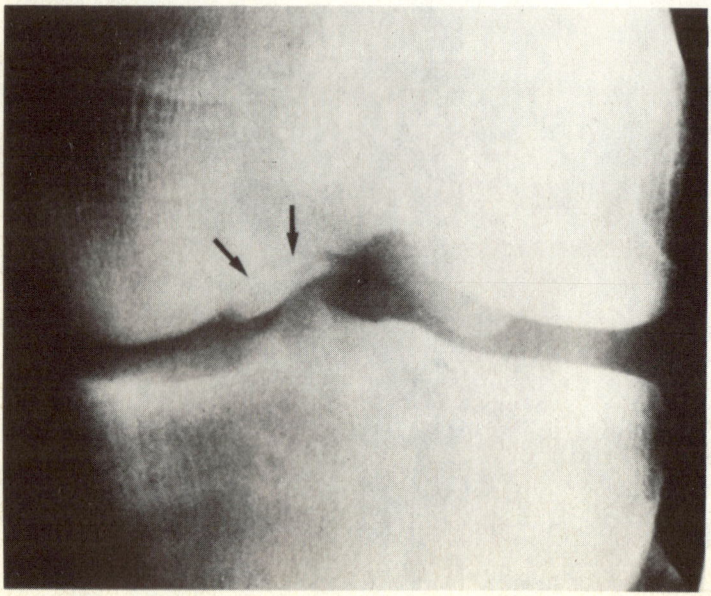

Plate 21. X-ray of a knee in a case of osteochondritis dissecans. The separating fragment of bone is arrowed.

present in 96 per cent of patients with ankylosing spondylitis. It is still uncertain how the HLA antigen influences disease susceptibility and there are a number of theories to account for the association. Perhaps it is not the HLA antigen itself, but a closely associated 'immume response' gene lying very nearby on the major histocompatability complex. According to this idea, people with HLA B27 will therefore react immunologically in a certain way when presented with an external stimulus, such as an infection, and spondylitis results. However, the actual evidence for infection in patients with ankylosing spondylitis is tenuous and details need not concern us closely. There are data which suggest the possibility of pelvic (genito-urinary) infection or chronic bowel inflammation as causative factors in a proportion of cases. Without too firm a basis of fact, our present concept is that some form of infection may act as a trigger mechanism in subjects who are genetically predisposed.

It is worth noting that the presence of HLA B27 is associated with the development of Reiter's syndrome (see page 56) and also with the reactive forms of arthritis which occasionally follow infections of the gut (to be discussed below): the latter represent a known association of infection triggering arthritis in HLA B27-positive susceptible subjects.

Treatment

Once the condition is diagnosed patients are encouraged to exercise in order to prevent postural deformities. The programme of exercises is quite extensive, involving breathing exercises, static contraction of abdominal and other trunk muscles, prone lying, active movements of the neck, shoulders, and arms, general postural discipline, and swimming. Instruction by a physiotherapist is therefore essential, after which the patient continues his exercises at home for the rest of his life. Spinal braces and other gadgets have little to recommend them and are rarely necessary.

In conjunction with exercises, medication reduces pain, stiffness, and inflammation. Phenylbutazone or indomethacin, taken regularly, are particularly useful drugs. Radiotherapy (X-ray treatment) eases pain and stiffness but has no known effect on the long-term course of the disease. It has rather fallen into disrepute after being shown to increase slightly the risks of developing leukaemia and marrow suppression: in any case most patients do well with the combination of exercise and an anti-inflammatory drug.

Rarely, in severe or advanced cases, surgical procedures designed to correct flexion deformities of the spine may be required; damaged hips can be treated by replacement arthroplasty.

Outlook

With proper management the outlook for patients with ankylosing spondylitis is reasonably favourable. Over 85 per cent of patients remain in their normal jobs, losing very little time from work. Extensive spinal rigidity need cause only little disability, provided that the vertebral column is maintained by appropriate exercises in a good functional position. Terrifying pictures in textbooks of men with ankylosing spondylitis almost bent double are to some extent a reflection of a pattern of treatment which was widespread about forty years ago, when the unfortunate victims were immobilized for many weeks in plaster beds or 'shells'. The muscles of the back became weakened and the patients became hunchbacks in which position the vertebrae would fuse.

Psoriatic arthritis

Psoriasis is a common chronic skin disorder of unknown cause, characterized by well-demarcated red scaly areas situated anywhere on the body, but commonly over the scalp, elbows, and knees. These areas are very variable in distribution, being in some patients extensive and unsightly and in others so trivial as to be detectable only by meticulous examination of the skin and nails.

Although rheumatoid arthritis and psoriasis, both being common diseases, may occasionally be found in the same individual, about 3 per cent of patients with psoriasis have a form of arthritis resembling, but usually distinguishable from, rheumatoid disease. Heredity is a prominent factor in the occurrence of psoriasis and psoriatic arthritis, although the exact mode of inheritance is not clear.

Features of psoriatic arthritis include involvement of the joints nearest to the finger tips, which are infrequently affected by rheumatoid arthritis (see Plate 15); tendon-sheath inflammation of one or two fingers giving a 'sausage-swelling' appearance; arthritis of only one or two joints, such as a single knee or wrist; and the development of sacro-iliitis or ankylosing spondylitis, often with the finding of HLA B27, though not so commonly as with ankylosing spondylitis in the absence of psoriasis. Psoriatic arthritis is usually a relatively mild disorder, compared with rheumatoid arthritis, but occasionally, in patients who are unfortunate enough to have extensive skin lesions, the joint disease too can be severe and disabling–so-called *arthritis mutilans*. Microscopic appearances of the synovial membrane are similar to those of rheumatoid arthritis, and erosions can be seen on X-ray, but rheumatoid factor is not found in the blood. Principles of treatment are similar to those of rheumatoid arthritis (Chapter 4).

Enteropathic arthritis

A few rather uncommon diseases of the intestine can sometimes be complicated by a form of inflammatory arthritis, to which the name 'enteropathic arthritis' has been given. The distressing disorder ulcerative colitis is accompanied in about 10 per cent of cases by arthritis which can resemble rheumatoid arthritis, but which more often involves only one joint–most often the knee or ankle–and which is seronegative. The bowel inflammation and the arthritis tend to flare up and subside together, and successful medical or surgical treatment of the colitis usually abolishes the joint symptoms. This suggests that the arthritis is in some way initiated by a factor within the gut, conceivably the absorption of antigenic material from the damaged mucous membrane of the intestine, followed by the formation of soluble antigen-antibody complexes which circulate in the blood and lead to joint inflammation. Sacro-iliitis and ankylosing spondylitis also occur in association with ulcerative colitis: HLA B27 is found in many of these patients, but not to the same extent as in ankylosing spondylitis alone. Similar patterns of joint disease complicate another inflammatory bowel disorder, Crohn's disease.

Joint disease occasionally follows some forms of gastro-intestinal infection. During infections with salmonella organisms (typhoid and paratyphoid fever) bacteria can reach a joint by way of the blood stream to produce a septic or infective arthritis. Perhaps more commonly–in about 3 per cent of cases–an acute arthritis involves a number of joints about 10 days after the infection and lasts for a few days. In such cases, however, the joint fluid itself is not infected; micro-organisms cannot be obtained from the joint fluid and it is sterile on culture. This type of arthritis, where joint inflammation follows an identified infection but the organism is not present in the joint, is called a reactive arthritis: antigenic bacterial products or complexes are again probably important causes. Most patients with reactive arthritis are HLA B27-positive.

Reiter's syndrome

This eponymous designation is an unsatisfactory term referring to a triad of urethritis (manifested by a purulent discharge from the urethra or urinary passage), arthritis, and conjunctivitis. The German army medical officer after whom the disease was named, who described the condition in 1916, was by no means the first to do so; Sir Benjamin Brodie of Guy's Hospital in London had reported it 100 years previously. Moreover, incomplete forms of the syndrome are often seen.

In the United Kingdom and North America most cases occur after extramarital sexual intercourse, urethritis resulting from direct infection. The nature of the agent responsible for the disease is uncertain. It is not the gonococcus (the microbe which causes gonorrhoea, an important and common form of urethritis) which can itself cause an infective type of arthritis, with blood-borne transport of the organism to the joint. A proportion of cases result from infection with an intracellular parasite called *Chlamydia trachomatis*. In many other parts of Europe, however, the clinical symptoms of Reiter's syndrome are preceded by an attack of bacillary dysentery. There are nevertheless patients from whom no history of venereal exposure or of diarrhoea can be obtained.

Most of the cases are young men. Joint symptoms commence about two weeks after the initial infection, urogenital or intestinal. It is a reactive arthritis, with sterile synovial fluid, characteristically acute and short lived, and usually confined to only a few joints, especially knees and ankles. Recovery is usually rapid, but sometimes there are recurrences and occasionally the disease takes on a chronic course with bone erosions, sacro-iliitis, and very rarely ankylosing spondylitis.

As with other forms of inflammatory polyarthritis, the erythrocyte sedimentation rate is elevated. A high proportion of cases–though not so many as with ankylosing spondylitis–possess the histocompatibility antigen HLA B27, particularly those with sacro-iliitis; by contrast, patients who acquire urethritis without the additional features of Reiter's syndrome show no increased prevalence of HLA B27. It therefore seems that a patient acquiring non-gonococcal urethritis who is HLA B27-positive has a high chance of developing Reiter's syndrome: the syndrome appears to result from the combination of a genetic predisposition–shown by B27 positivity–and an acquired urethral infection.

6

Osteoarthrosis

'Unfair wear and tear, my boy.' These words from an eminent surgeon constituted, as far as I can remember, my whole undergraduate training on the subject of osteoarthrosis (or osteoarthritis), one of the commonest of the rheumatic disorders. Estimates of its prevalence depend on diagnostic criteria, the methods of study employed, and the age of the population investigated. Moderate or severe changes were considered to be present in X-rays of the hands and feet in 11 per cent of persons in one large study, and abnormalities of mild degree can be seen in almost all individuals aged 65 or over. Although a proportion of these subjects do not have any symptoms, surveys in English industrial towns have shown that osteoarthrosis is an extremely common cause of loss of work in both men and women, confirmed by more specialized investigation among miners and dock-workers. Of the approximately 44 million days lost from work in Great Britain every year because of rheumatic complaints (about five times the number lost from industrial disputes) osteoarthrosis figures prominently: it is not just a problem of the aged.

No doubt man and his evolutionary ancestors have always suffered from osteoarthrosis, but it was only during the early years of the present century that it was delineated as an entity distinct from rheumatoid arthritis. The great German pathologist of the last century, Virchow, used the term arthritis deformans to describe both osteoarthrosis and rheumatoid disease. Another term, degenerative joint disease, is sometimes used synonymously with osteoarthrosis–it is not so much favoured nowadays, but has the merit of reminding us that the essential disorder is one of degenerative articular cartilage, contrasted with rheumatoid arthritis where the trouble commences with inflammation of the synovial membrane, to which cartilage erosion is secondary.

Osteoarthrosis is a disorder of diathrodial (synovial) joints characterized by localized splitting and fragmentation (fibrillation) of the articular cartilage. This process is accompanied or followed, to a variable degree, by hardening (sclerosis) of underlying bone; cysts in the bone, possibly formed by the pressure of joint fluid penetrating through cracks in the cartilage; progressive destruction of cartilage (so that the joint 'space' appears narrowed on X-ray); consequent exposure of the bone because of cartilage loss and bony outgrowths (osteophytes) forming as a reaction to the cartilage damage at the joint edges. It has been suggested that the initial lesion is essentially due to repetitive impulse loading causing microscopic fractures in the bone ends. Healing of these fractures causes bone sclerosis and stiffening of the bone, exposing the overlying cartilage to increased dynamic forces: in other words, the damage to cartilage results from previous damage and loss of elasticity in underlying bone.

Osteoarthrosis should not be viewed as a disease entity with a single cause. Various conditions–especially injury of one sort or another–predispose to its development; when such a condition can be identified the osteoarthrosis is said to be secondary to that condition. Otherwise osteoarthrosis is referred to as primary or idiopathic–which simply means that its causation in such cases is unknown. The whole problem of the biology of diarthrodial joints, their reaction to the loads placed upon them, remodelling of the bone, the nutrition of articular cartilage, joint lubrication, and the biochemical abnormalities causing, or caused by, osteoarthrosis are fields of intense research at present. Some interesting experimental work is being carried out but we do not yet have the answers.

Factors predisposing to osteoarthrosis

Age

No generalized, intrinsic, time-dependent deterioration of chondrocyte function has been demonstrated by numerous experimental studies, and articular cartilage can retain its normal appearance into old age. Nevertheless, the tensile strength and fatigue resistance of cartilage fall during adult life and the overall relation of age to osteoarthrosis is beyond question. Articular cartilage in many elderly people, however, remains remarkably healthy.

Mechanical abnormalities

Any event which alters the geometrical configuration of a joint, however slightly, can induce osteoarthrosis or accelerate its development. Such abnormalities may be the result of an inherited or congenital disorder of connective tissue, for example the group of conditions caused by defects of proteoglycan metabolism known as mucopolysaccharidoses and other rare diseases, in which bony deformities of the vertebrae and long bones lead to osteoarthrosis of neighbouring joints. Congenital dysplasia of the hip (dysplasia is a technical term meaning malformation), with or without actual dislocation, is a well-recognized precursor of secondary osteoarthrosis, and minor degrees are undoubtedly an important though often unrecognized cause. Veterinary surgeons are familiar with joint disease of this sort: well-known examples in the animal world include the congenital hip dysplasia found in highly in-bred golden retrievers.

Laxity of joint ligaments with abnormally mobile joints is a feature of certain rather rare congenital disorders, but joint laxity also occurs in otherwise healthy people. In one study investigators found hypermobile joints in 7 per cent of school children; most of us have friends or acquaintances who are 'double-jointed'. Joint mobility decreases with advancing age. People with lax joints are susceptible to transient joint effusions resulting from minor knocks and bangs and may go on to develop early osteoarthrosis, although in most such individuals the outlook is relatively good. Researchers are able to produce instability of a dog's knee joint by cutting one of the ligaments; osteoarthrosis rapidly follows. This procedure has been used to study the early biochemical changes of the disease.

Mechanical abnormalities resulting from injuries are a most important predisposing factor, either a single major injury or minor repetitive injuries sustained in certain occupations or sports. Examples include osteoarthrosis of the knees among coal-miners, osteoarthrosis of the fingers among cotton-mill workers and typists, and osteoarthrosis of the elbows and shoulders in pneumatic drill operators. Footballers are susceptible to osteoarthrosis of the knees and ankles and ballet dancers are reported to develop osteoarthrosis of the ankles, joints rarely affected in the general population. I have seen gross involvement of elbows and other joints in professional wrestlers and boxers.

Osteoarthrosis is also liable to occur when joints become badly aligned as a result of metabolic bone disease (such as rickets) or incorrectly set fractures.

Metabolic disease

Articular cartilage may be directly damaged as a consequence of a number of metabolic diseases. In gout, for example, it is weakened by the deposition of crystals of sodium urate; comparable deposition of calcium pyrophosphate occurs in chondrocalcinosis (these two forms of crystal synovitis are discussed in Chapter 7). In these and other metabolic disorders articular degeneration and osteoarthrosis are later features. The thickened cartilage in the rare endocrine disorder acromegaly is also liable to develop subsequent degenerative changes and osteoarthrosis.

We should here mention briefly the problem of obesity. Opinions differ regarding the influence of obesity, but there seems little doubt that excess body weight has a deleterious effect, at least as far as weight-bearing joints, particularly the knees, are concerned. Apart from the added load itself, it has been suggested that obese thighs force people to walk in a slightly bowlegged manner, this placing an extra strain on the inner (medial) compartment of the knee joint.

Inflammatory arthritis

We saw earlier how in rheumatoid arthritis and other forms of inflammatory polyarthritis the inflamed synovial membrane can erode articular cartilage and underlying bone. When this is severe the result may be a fusion of the bone ends by fibrous tissue (fibrous ankylosis), but osteoarthrosis may also be an end-result, with cartilage loss, bone sclerosis, and osteophyte formation. Indeed, there is good reason to suppose that many patients with osteoarthrosis have had a previous inflammatory type of arthritis, unbeknown to themselves.

As with rheumatoid arthritis, it is not believed that climate has any immediate influence on the development or course of osteoarthrosis, although exposure to cold and damp may well heighten awareness of pain from joints and similar connective structures. Nor does diet play any known part—except that over-eating makes a person fat, which is harmful.

Generalized osteoarthrosis

Osteoarthrosis, then, is often clearly a phenomenon secondary to some antecedent injury or disease. When such an underlying cause is not evident, the condition is termed primary, and when a number of joints are involved it is then referred to as primary generalized osteoarthrosis. This is extremely common. It involves particularly the joints nearest to the tips of the fingers, the bony enlargements of which are called Heberden's nodes (see Plate 2(b)). There is also painful loss of cartilage in the joints at the bases of the thumbs, the knees, and elsewhere. Primary generalized osteoarthrosis is found mainly in women over the age of 50 and tends to run in families.

Symptoms

From what has been written it will be appreciated that there is a wide variation in the symptoms of osteoarthrosis. The predominant symptom is pain, usually dull and persistent but worse on movement of the joint. It is sometimes difficult to understand such pain and its causation. Articular cartilage contains no nerves so that the early pathological changes found in cartilage are themselves painless. The deep layers of synovial membrane, joint capsule, and ligaments, on the other hand, are very sensitive but these structures are involved only relatively late in the course of the disease, when they may be damaged by minor degrees of injury due to joint instability and osteophyte formation. Again, the amount of pain experienced by different individuals with what appear to be similar degrees of joint change, as judged from clinical and radiological examination, is not at all constant. What to one person is no more than a trivial nuisance will to another be a degree of pain sufficient to seek medical advice. It is well recognized that reactions to a given pain stimulus vary a great deal, not only between different people but also in one person at different times, dependent on factors such as anxiety, worry, depression, and so on. This 'complaint threshold' is an important consideration in the assessment of a patient with osteoarthrosis (as, indeed, with any other rheumatic disease) and symptoms may well be compounded by psychological problems, such as the fear of a deforming and disabling arthritis; suitable reassurance can easily put this right, often with most satisfactory results.

Osteophyte formation causes bony swelling, easily detected in peripheral joints such as the joints of the fingers or the knees. The inflammatory soft tissue (synovial membrane) swelling and joint effusions of rheumatoid disease are generally only minor features of osteoarthrosis: when present they are due to injury to the synovial membrane. Heberden's nodes on the fingers, however, although usually painless little bony knobs, sometimes start off as acute, painful swellings, not unlike an attack of gout. It has indeed been suggested that such inflammatory features are due to the presence of apatite (calcium phosphate) microcrystals, analagous to the urate crystals which produce the acute gouty attack. Morning stiffness, another prominent symptom of rheumatoid arthritis, is mild or absent in osteoarthrosis. The erythrocyte sedimentation rate is normal and rheumatoid factors are not found in the blood.

Treatment

From what we have already seen it is evident that the disease processes taking place in the development of osteoarthrosis are to a considerable extent irreversible, certainly by the time that significant symptoms appear. This does not mean that symptoms may not improve, either spontaneously or with treatment, or that a great deal cannot be done to ease the situation, but it is useless to talk in terms of a 'cure', and a realistic assessment of the situation must be the first step in management.

Such an assessment may in itself be remarkably therapeutic. Countless middle-aged women consult their doctor with the first twinges of osteoarthrosis in the fingers, or the first signs of bony swelling. When the position is explained to them, their reaction is one of obvious relief. They will often confess the pain to be trivial and the mild deformity of the fingers, although by no means welcome, to be nevertheless of little consequence. Their anxiety has been that they might have rheumatoid arthritis, that they would go on to develop progressive and painful incapacity, and that they might be unable to meet their family responsibilities or continue their employment.

The doctor will advise on simple measures which may help. Joints and muscles should be kept warm, which means gloves for the hands and long-johns or thick tights under a pair of slacks when walking in cold weather. Pain from a hip joint is sometimes helped by asking a shoemaker to raise the heel on the affected side by a quarter of an inch. Much of what was written about physiotherapy in the treatment of rheumatoid arthritis (Chapter 4) applies here as well, particularly the vital importance of quadriceps exercises in maintaining the function of the knee joints. On the other hand over-use must be avoided and life must go on within the tolerance of damaged joints. Obesity should be corrected with a low-calorie diet.

Drug treatment is of secondary importance in osteoarthrosis and the more the patient can be encouraged to do without drugs the better: by the time pain becomes really severe a surgical consultation should be in the offing. Aspirin and other analgesics nevertheless have a part to play, and some patients do well on regular medication with phenylbutazone, indomethacin, or one of the other non-steroidal anti-inflammatory agents mentioned in Chapter 4. Gold salts, penicillamine, and corticosteroids are not used in the treatment of osteoarthrosis: a local steroid injection is occasionally helpful, particularly in the small joints at the base of the thumb.

Surgical treatment is indicated in severe osteoarthrosis of the hip. The exact indications for operation depend on a number of individual circumstances, such as the distance which can be walked, the degree of rest pain, and the age and general health of the patient. An operation known as osteotomy, in which the line of weight-bearing is altered by slightly displacing the upper part of the thigh bone in relation to its shaft, was formerly popular and is still carried out in some centres. Its exact value, however, is uncertain and total hip replacement (i.e. the insertion of an artificial hip) is now generally regarded as the operation of choice. It is safe and reliable; the functional life of modern prosthetic materials long outlasts that of their recipient; and the results in terms of pain relief and mobility are outstandingly good. The man or woman with osteoarthrosis has certain advantages as a candidate for surgery when compared to a patient with rheumatoid arthritis. Apart from the one or two joints seriously involved (osteoarthrosis may involve both hips) the rest of the musculoskeletal system is in good working order, and the general health is usually excellent, without the anaemia or other features of inflammation which may be found in subjects with rheumatoid disease.

Surgical replacement is also being used to an increasing extent in other joints, particularly the knees. Replacement operations in shoulders, elbows, and ankles are still in their early stages of development. Other surgical procedures are occasionally used, for example the fixation of a painful or unstable joint or the removal of loose pieces of bone. Osteoarthrosis involving the base of the great toe (hallux rigidus, hallux valgus), when causing symptoms, is also amenable to surgical treatment. Cosmetic operations are not to be recommended: surgical excision of Heberden's nodes is unsuccessful, because they grow again and look more unsightly than before.

As with other chronic rheumatic disorders, many less conventional types of therapy have been attempted, but none have been shown to give any benefit. They include acupuncture, the injection of silicone oil into the joint, and the administration of an extract of calf rib cartilage and bone marrow called Rumalon.

Outlook

The outlook in mild osteoarthrosis, particularly primary generalized osteoarthrosis, is usually good with regard to functional capacity. Heberden's nodes, for example, are either painless from the onset or become so and although they persist indefinitely as rather unsightly bony knobs only the finest actions of the fingers are impaired. Again, involvement of the joints at the base of the thumb can be painful and may weaken the grip a little, but serious incapacity is rare. On the other hand, a major joint, especially if weight-bearing, may be quite another matter: painful and disabling joint degeneration is an unwelcome legacy from an injury to a knee or ankle many years previously and osteoarthrosis of the hip is a cruel cause of crippling in the elderly. Even here, however, sequential studies have shown that many patients maintain a steady functional state, without progressive deterioration, over a period of years. Fortunately, too, for those in whom the disease is progressive modern surgery has much to offer.

7

Gout and other related forms of arthritis

'Metabolism' can be defined as the processes by which nutritive material from broken-down foodstuffs is built up into various forms of living matter (anabolism) or by which living matter is itself broken down into simpler substances (catabolism), with release of energy. Countless biochemical reactions are involved. Diseases involving these processes can affect the joints and connective tissue: in the last chapter we saw how some inherited metabolic defects could cause abnormalities of articular cartilage leading to osteoarthrosis. Most such disorders, however, though numerous, are rare and need no description in this book.

Although the part played by crystalline deposits of sodium urate in the acute attack of gout was suggested during the last century, it has only been within the past 20 years that their detection in joint fluid has become a standard diagnostic procedure. They have come to be easily recognized under the microscope as needle-shaped crystals, rather variable in size (between 2 and 20 micrometres in length) but regular in shape and showing certain optical characteristics (negative birefringence) when viewed under a polarizing microscope. The details of these optical features need not concern us.

It was soon realized that another type of crystal could also be associated with an acute inflammatory reaction in a joint, distinguishable from urate by its rather irregular shape and positive sign of birefringence; it was subsequently identified by crystallographic techniques as calcium pyrophosphate dihydrate. The acute synovitis caused by these crystals resembled gout in many ways and was therefore called 'pseudogout'. Calcification of articular cartilage, or chondrocalcinosis, is usually seen on X-ray examination and it is by this name that the condition is usually known.

There are therefore two main types of crystal synovitis that we shall discuss in this chapter: gout (sodium urate) and chondrocalcinosis (calcium pyrophosphate), both are quite common rheumatic diseases. Some other metabolic disorders will also be mentioned.

Arthritis and Rheumatism

Gout

Gout is a disease with a strong tendency to run in families. It is seen predominantly in adult men, characterized by episodes of acute arthritis, and later also by chronic damage to joints and other structures. It is caused essentially by hyperuricaemia, an excess of uric acid in the blood and tissues. With increasing knowledge of uric acid metabolism it has become evident that there are many factors which can influence the development of hyperuricaemia and hence of gout. Gouty arthritis may therefore be regarded as the end-result of a number of different biochemical processes, which will be outlined later in the chapter. The term primary gout is used when hyperuricaemia is due principally to an inherited metabolic abnormality and secondary gout when it is largely the result of an acquired disease or some known environmental factor. First, however, I shall describe the salient features of the gout syndrome.

Estimates of prevalence obtained from epidemiological surveys vary widely. From a recent study in Framingham, U.S.A., came figures of 28 per 1000 for men and 4 per 1000 for women, but such figures can be taken as general approximations only. The prevalence of hyperuricaemia and gout is known to vary between populations and there appears little doubt that it can change, owing to environmental and particularly dietary factors, in the same population over quite a short time. For example, it is generally held that gout is much more common in Europe than it was during the Second World War; it is seen quite frequently today in Spain, where it was almost unknown during the Civil War.

Symptoms

People who develop gout have usually lived for many years, unbeknown to themselves, with a raised plasma level of uric acid (asymptomatic hyperuricaemia) until eventually crystals of sodium urate, precipitated in a joint, provoke a sudden tissue reaction which leads to the first attack of acute gouty arthritis. Each acute attack lasts for only a short period, being followed by intervals of widely varying duration during which there is again complete freedom from symptoms (intercritical gout) although hyperuricaemia persists. Some people may have only one or two episodes of acute gouty arthritis in the whole of their lives, while others suffer repeated attacks of increasing duration, severity, and frequency, one running into another and involving joint after joint. In time some joints no longer return to their normal state; deposits of urate (tophi) form around the joints and elsewhere; and the patient has entered the stage of chronic tophaceous gouty arthritis.

Blood levels of uric acid are generally higher in men than in women, and this is reflected by a predominance of gouty arthritis among men. Of 354 patients with gout studied some years ago by Dr. Rodney Grahame and myself, 311 (88 per cent) were men and 43 (12 per cent) women.

Acute gouty arthritis is an inflammatory reaction caused by the presence of sodium urate crystals within a joint. It starts, usually in a single joint, as a sensation of discomfort developing over a period of hours into pain which can be very severe indeed, an excruciating torment in fact. Attacks often commence at night, awakening the unfortunate victim from his sleep. The affected joint becomes reddened, shiny, swollen, and exquisitely tender (Plate 16); in the larger joints, such as the knee, an inflammatory effusion accumulates. The weight of a sheet on the foot may be intolerable and the apprehensive sufferer will hardly allow an examining hand to approach the painful limb, let alone palpate it. Unless terminated by colchicine or other drugs the attack may last for several days or weeks, but the condition of the joint eventually returns to normal.

The joint at the base of the great toe is involved in over 70 per cent of cases, followed in frequency by the foot, ankle, knee, fingers, and wrist. Attacks usually occur spontaneously, but may be precipitated by trauma, a blow on the knee or wrist, for example, being followed several hours later by an attack of gout in that joint. Gout also tends to occur during or after illnesses such as pneumonia, and sometimes follows surgical operations.

Chronic tophaceous gouty arthritis, due to the deposition of solid urate in relation to articular structures, leads to destructive arthritis with secondary osteoarthrosis. It usually follows repeated acute attacks but can develop insidiously in a previously unaffected joint. Such permanent changes are often prominent in the joints of the fingers (Plate 5c). The skin overlying the tophaceous deposits becomes thinned, and through it can sometimes be seen the white mass of underlying sodium urate, which may later discharge itself as the skin breaks and ulcerates. About one-fifth of patients with gout develop tophi and permanent joint damage; the figure may have been higher in the past and is no doubt falling with modern methods of controlling uric acid levels.

Tophi are found elsewhere than in immediate relation to joints. They are particularly common on the cartilages of the ear lobe, where they form small white excrescences about 1–4 millimetres across (see Plate 17). Uric acid or sodium urate may also be deposited in various internal organs; this is rarely of clinical importance except in the kidneys where uric acid stones may form in a proportion of gout patients: they are usually small and passed in the urine without too much difficulty, although they can cause the painful condition known as renal colic. Various forms of kidney disease and high blood pressure are undoubtedly frequent in patients with gout although in any one individual it may be difficult to establish the exact sequence of events which has taken place—for example, whether deposition of uric acid has caused kidney damage, or kidney disease has impaired the excretion of uric acid.

The clinical features of gout are very distinctive in a typical case. A raised level of uric acid in the blood is necessary to confirm the diagnosis although hyperuricaemia in itself does not establish a diagnosis of gout, since many people have a raised level of uric acid without suffering from gouty arthritis. The identification of urate crystals from an involved joint or from a tophus is a most useful diagnostic aid (see Plate 18).

Causes of high uric acid levels in the blood

Although there are a number of local factors, as yet incompletely understood, which lead to the deposition of urate in solid crystalline form, the development of gouty arthritis must be regarded as primarily related to the degree and duration of hyperuricaemia—an elevated blood level of uric acid. The prevalence of gout is high in populations (such as the Maoris of New Zealand) whose uric acid levels are above those found in Europe; epidemiological surveys have shown a correlation between the height of the serum urate value and the prevalence of gout.

Now for a little organic chemistry. Uric acid is the end-product of purine metabolism in man. Purines comprise a class of chemical substances with a certain molecular ring configuration; they are essential constituents of cell nuclei. Purines are derived in the body either preformed from the diet, from the breakdown of tissue nucleic acids, or by a process of chemical synthesis from simple precursor substances. Most mammals possess an enzyme called uricase, which can disrupt the purine ring and break down uric acid to other end-products of metabolism, but late in the course of mammalian evolution the enzyme has been lost, so that man and the higher primates have to excrete uric acid as such. Most uric acid is excreted into the urine by the kidneys although some passes into the intestine.

It will therefore be apparent that the plasma level of uric acid can be raised by a number of factors, inborn or environmental, acting either alone or in combination. These involve basically (1) an increased metabolic rate of uric acid formation; (2) a decreased rate of excretion by the kidney; and (3) other factors associated with hyperuricaemia and gout, the exact mechanisms of which are uncertain. During the past few years a great deal has been learnt about these various processes. An increased production of uric acid, for example, is found when there is an exaggerated turnover of nucleic acid purines in diseases –such as leukaemia–accompanied by excessive cellular breakdown; while of exceptional interest, though rare, are various genetic abnormalities in the regulation of certain enzymes concerned with purine metabolism. We have also discovered numerous factors which can regulate the amount of uric acid excreted by the kidney. They vary widely, ranging from starvation and alcoholic intoxication to lead poisoning and a number of drugs (for example, diuretics) which are in common use. Also related to uric acid levels are other factors such as race, sex, age, and body weight. Weight reduction in an obese person will lower his blood level of uric acid. There tends to be a positive correlation between levels of uric acid and those of certain lipids, particularly triglycerides, and the problem of the relationship between uric acid and cardiovascular disease remains to be clarified. There may be some association between hyperuricaemia and coronary artery disease, but this is to a large extent dependent upon other associated factors such as body weight and high blood pressure. Hyperuricaemia in the absence of such associations does not appear to be a coronary risk factor.

In most patients with gout, however, as we see them in our clinics, the cause or causes of their raised uric acid level remains uncertain. Some can be shown to be 'over-producers' of uric acid while many are 'under-excretors'. To such inborn errors of metabolism are added in many instances the effects of external agents, particularly food (with regard to both its purine and calorie content), alcoholic liquors, and drugs.

Treatment

It is nowadays possible to control both the inflammation of acute gouty arthritis and the level of uric acid in the blood with a facility which is considerably in advance of our understanding of some of the pathological and physiological features of the disorder. The time is long past since severe acute attacks and tophus formation progressed in the face of tedious dietary restriction. Proper handling of appropriate drugs should keep most patients entirely free of symptoms.

Treatment of acute gout is directed towards relief of inflammation as rapidly as possible. Control of uric acid itself plays no part in the treatment of acute gouty arthritis and attempts to lower the blood level at this stage may well prolong the episode. A number of drugs are available. Colchicine is the time-honoured remedy, effective but tending to cause diarrhoea, nausea, or vomiting. Newer drugs such as phenylbutazone, indomethacin, or naproxen are therefore usually preferred.

When an acute attack has been terminated the question of long-term management is considered, with particular reference to lowering the serum uric acid. This is a decision of some importance, because once started such treatment must be continued regularly and indefinitely. It is therefore necessary for both doctor and patient to be convinced of its necessity. Indications for lowering the serum urate vary slightly with individual cases, but treatment should usually be commenced in one of the following situations:

1 Gout with chronic joint changes or tophi.
2 Frequent acute attacks.
3 Evidence of kidney damage.
4 Gout accompanied by a considerably elevated serum level of uric acid–8 mg/100 ml (480 μmol/l) or over–because the disease is then usually progressive, in terms of both frequency of attacks and the development of chronic joint damage.

In the absence of these criteria–for example following one or two mild attacks with only a moderately elevated uric acid–there is nothing to be lost by awaiting the course of events for a while. In particular, long-term treatment should not be started when there is any doubt about diagnosis. A rare exception is the patient who presents with atypical joint symptoms in the presence of hyperuricaemia, when it may be justifiable to lower the uric acid for some months as a form of therapeutic trial. Such situations are very unsatisfactory, however, and such a step should not be taken before the fullest possible investigation has been carried out. Sometimes a patient with a symptom which is fairly obviously *not* due to gout (such as a frozen shoulder or osteoarthrosis of the hip) is nevertheless subjected to an estimation of the serum uric acid and coincident hyperuricaemia treated with urate lowering drugs, which are then both unnecessary and symptomatically ineffective. This condition of 'non-gout' is very common today.

If it is decided to lower the serum uric acid, this may be done either with drugs which increase the excretion of uric acid from the kidneys or with allopurinol. Drugs in the first group include probenecid (Benemid) and sulphinpyrazone (Anturan). Allopurinol (Zyloric) lowers the uric acid level in quite a different manner, by inhibiting its formation. Although acute attacks of gout may remain troublesome during the early weeks or months of treatment, they eventually become less frequent and eventually terminate altogether, provided that the level of uric acid has been consistently lowered by regular medication in adequate dosage (Fig. 4).

Other measures in gout are of secondary importance. Severe dietary restriction is unnecessary, though it probably wise to observe moderation with regard to alcohol and high-purine foods, which include

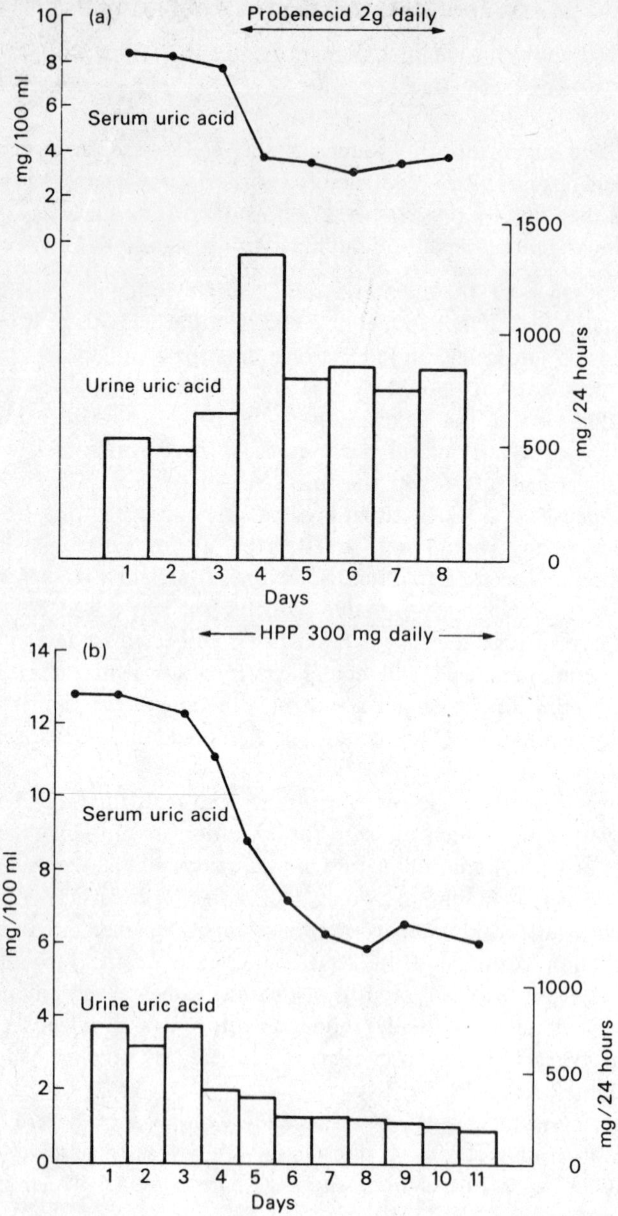
(a)
Probenecid 2g daily
Serum uric acid
mg/100 ml
10
8
6
4
2
0
Urine uric acid
1500
1000
500
0
mg/24 hours
1 2 3 4 5 6 7 8
Days
HPP 300 mg daily
(b)
14
12
10
8
6
4
2
0
mg/100 ml
Serum uric acid
Urine uric acid
1000
500
0
mg/24 hours
1 2 3 4 5 6 7 8 9 10 11
Days

sweetbreads, liver, kidney, fish-roe, and tinned fish. Gouty subjects tend to be overweight, and this may require attention. As already noted, weight reduction may itself lower the plasma urate level and correct mild degrees of hyperuricaemia. Large tophi can be removed surgically if necessary, but again the serum urate should be satisfactorily controlled beforehand.

A final problem is that of asymptomatic hyperuricaemia. In these days of health screening and multi-channel biochemical investigation it occasionally happens that a serum uric acid estimation is carried out on a person with no history of gout. The problem then arises as to the action to be taken, if any, if the level is elevated. There is no doubt, from epidemiological studies referred to above, that hyperuricaemia carries a proportionate risk of gouty arthritis, but this can be dealt with when and if it occurs. Rather more concern may be felt about the possible development of kidney or cardiac disease. A person with hyperuricaemia should be given a full clinical assessment as for a patient with overt gout, but in the absence of any other abnormality there is no evidence that lowering the plasma rate will have a preventative action with regard to anything except gouty arthritis or, rarely (presumably), kidney stones. It is therefore generally felt that mild degrees of hyperuricaemia may be observed judiciously; opinions with regard to higher levels of uric acid–say above 8 mg/100 ml (480 μmol/l)–differ, but sympathy can be felt for the view that such people, particularly if over-producers, should be given the benefit of the doubt and treated with allopurinol.

Chondrocalcinosis

The condition of chondrocalcinosis can exist without any symptoms and cartilage calcification can be seen in X-rays of elderly people who have never had any joint pain. The presence of pyrophosphate crystals within the synovial cavity, however, can produce acute syn-

---

Fig. 4. Reduction of serum uric acid by (a) 2 g probenecid daily and (b) allopurinol (HPP, hydroxypyrazolopyrimidine). Probenecid increases the excretion of uric acid, shown by the columns. Allopurinol inhibits the formation of uric acid and urinary uric acid therefore falls. (See opposite.)

ovitis very similar to gout: the affected joint becomes suddenly painful, warm, red, swollen, and tender. The knee is most commonly involved, followed by the wrist and other large joints: the great toe is only rarely affected.

Deposition of calcium pyrophosphate may also cause a more chronic type of arthritis involving small joints, rather like rheumatoid arthritis. It is also seen in association with osteoarthrosis, of which it appears to be a cause.

Diagnosis may not be possible on initial clinical examination, but the radiological appearance of chondrocalcinosis (see Plate 19) and the detection of pyrophosphate crystals when fluid is removed from the joint soon clarify the position.

What are the factors leading to deposition of calcium pyrophosphate? We have to confess our ignorance. Unlike gout, where a raised level of uric acid in the blood is a necessary prequisite for the precipitation of urate crystals, there is so far no evidence of a systemic disease or generalized metabolic defect in most patients with chondrocalcinosis. It is true that conditions in which the calcium level in the blood is elevated–as, for example, in overactivity of the parathyroid glands–may lead to chondrocalcinosis, but this is very uncommon: the calcium level is nearly always found to be normal.

It should also be added that the crystal story is probably even more complicated. Another type of calcific deposition (calcium phosphate or apatite) occurs in relation to joint capsules and tendon sheaths where it can produce localized painful conditions.

Other types of metabolic arthritis

Endocrine disorders

Diseases of the endocrine or ductless glands of the body can sometimes produce articular disease: the rarity and vague symptomatology of these disorders often lead to misdiagnosis.

It has just been pointed out that excess activity of the parathyroid glands (hyperparathyroidism) raises the calcium level of the blood and predisposes to chondrocalcinosis. In the process, calcium is withdrawn from bone with the production of lesions which can sometimes closely resemble rheumatoid erosions.

There are other endocrine diseases with rheumatological manifestations. In acromegaly, overactivity of the pituitary gland leads to overgrowth of soft tissues and cartilage with subsequent osteoarthrosis and joint destruction. Overgrowth of subcutaneous tissue at the wrist causes pressure on the median nerve and the carpal tunnel syndrome (Chapter 11, page 112).

Hypothyroidism, or myxoedema, the state of underactivity of the thyroid gland, causes a fall in metabolic rate with physical and intellectual slowing, tiredness, and weakness. Rheumatic symptoms occur but tend to be ill-defined. True synovial swelling and effusion are rare, but muscle cramps and skeletal pain are relatively common and pressure on the median nerve in the wrist by swollen myxoedematous tissue can again cause the carpal tunnel syndrome.

Metabolic bone disease

As mentioned above, hyperparathyroidism causes withdrawal of calcium from bone and destructive lesions underlying the articular cartilage.

Osteomalacia is a condition where calcification of the framework of bone is defective, due to deficiency of vitamin D (either dietary or resulting from impaired intestinal absorption), calcium deficiency, or certain forms of kidney disease. Joint disease as such does not occur, but a combination of diffuse bone pain and accompanying muscle weakness can produce a clinical picture rather resembling generalized arthritis. The childhood counterpart of osteomalacia is *rickets*, where severe deformities of developing bones and joints are a feature.

By contrast osteoporosis is a reduction of total bone mass, the bony framework itself being normally calcified. It occurs in localized forms as, for example, when a limb is immobilized or in proximity to an inflamed joint. Generalized osteoporosis occurs in elderly people, particularly women; in some forms of malnutrition; and in the presence of an excess of adrenal hormones, either as a consequence of disease or following the administration of steroid hormones in large dosage. Bone pain is due to collapse and fracture.

Pregnancy, the contraceptive pill, and the menopause

The symptoms of rheumatoid arthritis are sometimes temporarily suppressed during the later months of pregnancy, an observation which 30 years ago led Dr. Philip Hench of the Mayo Clinic to investigate the use of cortisone to treat rheumatoid arthritis. On the other hand, pregnancy, which imposes bichemical, physiological, mechanical, and psychological stresses, is sometimes accompanied by its own musculo-skeletal syndromes. These include low back pain and pelvic pain associated with relaxation and separation of the pubic bones.

Joint pains and rheumatic symptoms occasionally occur in women taking oral contraceptive preparations. They tend to be mild and cause no disability.

The term 'menopausal arthritis' has no firm pathological basis. Of course the symptoms of rheumatoid arthritis or osteoarthrosis may coincide with the change of life but there is no special form of arthritis associated with the menopause.

Other metabolic disorders

These include the hyperlipoproteinaemias, where excess of cholesterol or other lipids can lead to deposition of fats in bones and joints with the appearance of arthritis; haemochromatosis, where abnormal deposition of iron leads to chondrocalcinosis and joint damage; ochronosis, where a rare inherited metabolic disorder is shown by deposition of pigment in cartilage and intervertebral discs; Wilson's disease, in which a congenital disorder of copper metabolism presents itself predominantly by damage to the brain and liver, but where several types of joint abnormality are recognized; and many others.

The multiplicity and complexity of the various types of metabolic diseases and their effects upon bones and joints emphasize yet again the hopeless inadequacy of terms such as 'arthritis' and 'rheumatism' as diagnostic labels in themselves.

8

Rheumatic diseases in childhood

There is a tendency to associate rheumatic diseases with the elderly, and certainly, as we have already seen, many of the common rheumatic disorders occur predominantly in middle age or later life. They can, however, occur in childhood, and their individual impact on child and parents is then of course considerable in terms of suffering, disability, and anxiety. Fortunately, childhood rheumatic diseases are rare: rheumatic fever has virtually disappeared from all except the poorest countries of the world and the outlook for the child with chronic forms of arthritis has improved considerably with modern standards of management.

In this chapter a description of rheumatic fever will be presented to the reader, because it has been a common disease within living memory and remains so in developing countries. This will be followed by an account of the various forms of juvenile chronic arthritis.

Rheumatic fever

Rheumatic fever ('acute rheumatism') is characterized by fever, polyarthritis (that is, inflammation of a number of joints), and carditis (that is, inflammation of the heart). Unlike rheumatoid arthritis and many other rheumatic diseases the external cause is known beyond any doubt whatsoever; it is preceding infection by a microbe known as the Group A beta-haemolytic streptococcus. The declining incidence in modern times of streptococcal infection is responsible for the disappearance of rheumatic fever, one of the most dramatic epidemiological events of the past 50 years. Formerly among the commonest of the serious diseases of childhood, it was reported as recently as 1928 to fill 25 per cent of the beds at the Great Ormond Street Children's Hospital in London. By 1930, however, it was already referred to by Dr. J. A. Glover, Medical Officer of the Board of Education, as an 'obsolescent' disease. At the Canadian Red Cross Memorial Hospital,

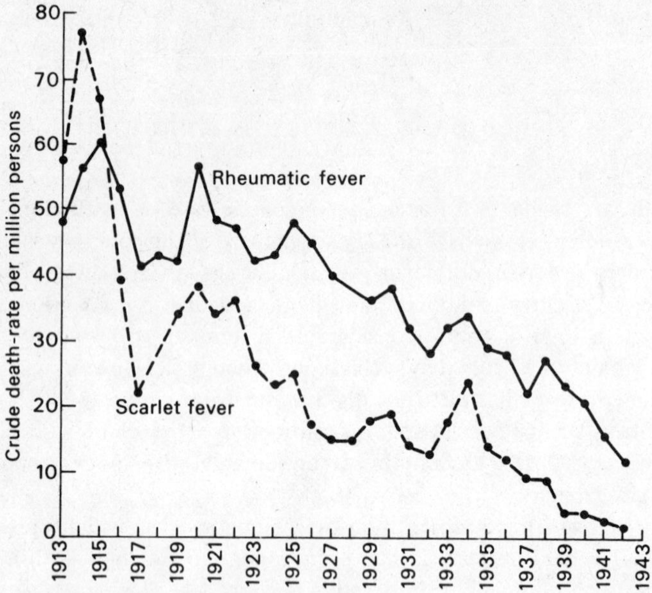

Fig. 5. Declining death-rates of rheumatic fever and scarlet fever (Glover (1943). By courtesy of the Editor of *The Lancet*).

Taplow, the leading centre in England for the study and treatment of all forms of rheumatic diseases in childhood, admissions for rheumatic fever fell from 146 in 1942 to 4 in 1973.

A decrease in the severity of the disease has also taken place, as shown by its decreasing mortality rate, which has run in parallel with that of scarlet fever, another post-streptococcal illness (Fig. 5). These figures, however, do not include deaths from chronic rheumatic heart disease, which may occur many years after the acute illness.

It should again be emphasized that the disease remains common and virulent in developing countries. In Egypt, for example, near the Pyramids, a short distance from Cairo, there is a 600-bed hospital exclusively for young people with rheumatic fever and rheumatic heart disease. It is a beautiful building, a model of cleanliness and efficiency, where all aspects of treatment, including rehabilitation in sheltered employment, are carefully carried out by Professor Abdin and her colleagues.

The causative role of Group A beta-haemolytic streptococci is based on several pieces of evidence. For example, studies of individual patients and epidemics have shown that outbreaks of rheumatic fever follow streptococcal infection, usually a sore throat, and streptococcal antibody levels are raised in patients with rheumatic fever, indeed to a greater extent than in uncomplicated streptococcal infection. On the other hand, immediate damage to joints and heart by the presence of the microbe is unlikely: organisms are not found in the actual lesions of the disease and doses of penicillin sufficient to eradicate them do not cut short an established attack of rheumatic fever. Again, streptococcal infection is common but only a minority of victims develop rheumatic fever, so that other factors must be involved.

From the work of Kaplan in the U.S.A. and others, using human clinical and experimental animal data, it appears that an 'autoimmune' mechanism may be operative, and that in certain susceptible subjects an immunological reaction mounted against an invading streptococcus may, because of molecular similarities, also occur against heart tissue, notably that of the heart, with consequent tissue damage.

Over 60 years ago Dr. Robert Hutchinson commented that rheumatic fever was 'essentially a working class disease', and associations have been demonstrated with social grade, income, and overcrowding. The last is probably of particular importance, since it would predispose to both the frequency and severity of streptococcal infection. The decline in rheumatic fever, therefore, may be attributed to improving socio-economic conditions rather than to any purely medical measures. A disease predominantly of children, rheumatic fever is very uncommon before the age of 4 years, reaching a peak incidence about the age of 8. It is nowadays hardly ever seen in adults except during epidemics.

Following a sore throat there is a 'silent interval' lasting from several days to a few weeks. Then follows a rather variable picture, ranging from an acute illness with fever, sweating, and arthritis to mild complaints of lassitude and vague limb pains. The joint pain is characteristically 'flitting', involving a single joint at a time, often with quite intense pain and swelling. Unlike rheumatoid arthritis, where superficial layers of the synovial membrane show an inflammatory reaction, the areas of inflammation in rheumatic fever affect mainly the deeper tissues of the joint capsule. Joint involvement of this sort continues for some weeks but nearly always settles down with complete recovery. Other transient signs include a skin rash and the presence of nodules under the skin: the latter tend to be smaller than the nodules of rheumatoid arthritis and the appearance of the nodular tissue under the microscope is rather different.

It is the heart, however, which is the main cause for concern and during the course of rheumatic fever the physician will repeatedly examine the child for signs of inflammation in cardiac tissue—be it in the inner lining of the heart, the valves, the cardiac muscle, or the pericardium, the outer sheath of the heart. In some cases there may be no signs of carditis, while in others they may be restricted to minor changes in the electrocardiogram. More severe involvement can produce scarring of the valves leading to heart failure in later years, or occasionally death during the acute illness itself. Rheumatic fever unfortunately tends to recur, fresh heart damage taking place with each recurrence.

Another accompaniment of rheumatic fever is Sydenham's chorea ('St. Vitus's dance'), with its involuntary and unco-ordinated muscular movements. It tends to be a late complication, and varies in severity from barely perceptible grimacing and inattention to severe and even fatal cases.

Laboratory tests of value in the diagnosis and management of rheumatic fever include the erythrocyte sedimentation rate, which is invariably abnormal during active phases of the disease, and tests for streptococcal antibodies in the blood, particularly the antistreptolysin O titre: the latter is a sign of preceding streptococcal infection but not necessarily of rheumatic fever. The clinical diagnosis of rheumatic fever is often a very difficult exercise: it can mimic, or be mimicked by, many other conditions such as acute appendicitis or osteomyelitis. Particularly important is the avoidance of a cardiac neurosis in child or parents due to the presence of an innocent heart murmur.

The importance of sociological factors in the prevention of rheumatic fever has already been stressed. The acute illness is treated by limiting the work of the heart by physical rest and the use of anti-inflammatory drugs, particularly salicylates (aspirin) and corticosteroid hormones, during the acute stage of the disease. Recurrences are prevented by long-term prophylaxis with penicillin or sulphonamides.

Juvenile chronic arthritis

Chronic (that is, protracted) arthritis is rare in children. Towards the end of the last century Dr. G. F. Still of Great Ormond Street Children's Hospital, London, described a number of such patients; chronic arthritis in children came thus to be known as 'Still's disease'. The modern tendency is to restrict this term to the type of illness emphasized by Still–joint pain and swelling, often with high fever and prominent lymph glands. There are certainly several different types of polyarthritis in children, as in adults: our ideas about nomenclature and classification are hampered by complete ignorance of their underlying causes.

As recommended at a recent workshop sponsored by the European League against Rheumatism and the World Health Organization in Oslo in 1977, the term 'juvenile chronic arthritis' is now considered to be the preferred term to cover this heterogeneous group of conditions.

Adult-type rheumatoid arthritis

This group forms only a small proportion of the whole. The clinical picture is similar to that of rheumatoid arthritis in adults (Chapter 3), with symmetrical polyarthritis, erosion of cartilage and bone, the presence of IgM rheumatoid factor in the blood and sometimes nodules and vasculitis.

Juvenile ankylosing spondylitis

Ankylosing spondylitis has been described in Chapter 5. It can start in childhood and such cases form a small but important group of children with chronic arthritis. Their clinical diagnosis may be difficult at first; the lesions of spondylitis or of inflammation of the sacro-iliac joints may not be apparent, the child (usually a boy) presenting himself with arthritis of one or several peripheral joints. The presence of the histocompatibility antigen HLA B27 or a family history of spondylitis may be an important clue. As with the adult disease, the course may be punctuated by episodes of inflammation of the eyes (iritis) with acute pain and redness.

Still's disease

This clinical pattern is truly 'juvenile', its occurrence in adults being unusual. Apart from pain and swelling in the joints, systemic or constitutional features are prominent, particularly a high swinging temperature, enlargement of the lymph glands and occasionally the spleen, and a characteristic patchy measles-like rash which tends to come and go with the fever. Indeed, the fever and general illness may come on long before the joint symptoms, a very difficult diagnostic situation. This is illustrated by the following case history:

A 14-year old boy recently became ill with a high temperature lasting for many months. He was extremely unwell and had lost weight. Extensive investigation in hospital failed to elucidate the cause of the fever, and an exploring abdominal operation (to search for some underlying malignant condition) was proposed. Before this could be undertaken, however, the correct diagnosis was indicated by the appearance of the typical rash of Still's disease, followed a little later by pain and swelling in the joints. The boy became completely free of symptoms on treatment with the steroid hormone prednisolone: it was later possible to reduce the dosage and eventually to discontinue the drug altogether.

Two further varieties of Still's disease, probably separate entities from each other and from the systemic type just described, consist of a group with multiple joint involvement and a further group with involvement of only one or a few joints, sometimes with the insidious onset of chronic iritis (emphasizing the need for expert ophthalmic examination in all cases of juvenile arthritis) and the presence in the blood of antinuclear antibodies. These antibodies are often a feature of the apparently unrelated inflammatory disease of connective tissue known as systemic lupus erythematosus (Chapter 10). Patients with

Still's disease have a raised erythrocyte sedimentation rate but do not possess IgM rheumatoid factor.

Juvenile forms of other types of inflammatory polyarthritis

Such conditions as psoriatic arthritis, or the arthritis accompanying inflammatory bowel disease (Chapter 5) can start in childhood, as can polyarthritis associated with other inflammatory disorders of connective tissue (Chapter 10).

The overall prognosis in juvenile chronic arthritis is relatively favourable compared with that of adults, though this depends to some extent on the type of involvement: for example the outlook in children with IgM rheumatoid factor tends to be rather worse than those without. One study showed that 83 per cent of the cases were able to work 15 years after onset.

A serious and often fatal complication–though fortunately uncommon–is the immunological tissue reaction known as amyloid. Infection is another cause of death. Arthritis in children can also influence the growth of bone, resulting sometimes in generalized growth retardation or localized developmental anomalies.

The principles of general management in juvenile chronic arthritis are similar to those in adult rheumatoid disease (Chapter 4). They are basically simple enough but often difficult in practice, depending on close rapport with the child, prolonged parental co-operation, and adequate supporting services. Avoidance of deformity and maintainance of function by correct physical treatment are crucial: flexion contractures of wrists and knees can otherwise develop with alarming rapidity. The principles of drug treatment are also similar. Aspirin is very useful, controlling both symptoms and the high temperature of Still's disease. Corticosteroids, in addition to their other disadvantages, tend to suppress growth, although this can sometimes be overcome by dosage on alternate days. Gold, and possibly penicillamine, have their parts to play in selected cases, and surgical treatment, too, is occasionally indicated, although some types of operation, such as joint replacement, are usually best deferred until growth has ceased. All these therapeutic measures have to be undertaken in association with the provision of psychological support and schooling. The treatment of juvenile chronic arthritis is indeed a matter for the experienced specialist.

This chapter has been confined to a discussion of rheumatic fever and juvenile chronic arthritis. There are many other types of joint disease which can occur in childhood including those due to infections (bacterial or viral), Henoch-Schonlein purpura, leukaemia, and the inflammatory disorders of connective tissue. They are not confined to children, however, and are therefore included in the following two chapters.

9

Other forms of arthritis

Most of the major forms of arthritis have now been discussed. Numerous other types of joint disease nevertheless remain: many of them need not be described, either because of their complexity or rarity, but some of the more important should be mentioned.

Infective arthritis

Infectious agents are known to play a prominent role in many of the rheumatic diseases, and possibly do so in others, but the actual mechanisms by which they produce tissue damage are variable. Easiest to understand is the situation where micro-organisms gain direct access to a joint—for example, through the blood-stream—and the terms infective, septic, or suppurative arthritis usually refer to this immediate damage by a microbe. Secondly, microbial or viral antigens may appear in a joint at some stage following the infective process: tissue damage may be caused by immune complexes (Chapter 3, p. 27) formed by union of these antigens with corresponding antibodies. Thirdly, as we discussed in Chapter 5, there is a syndrome termed 'reactive arthritis' where, in a susceptible individual, invasion of the body by certain types of organisms, particularly those causing infection of the gut or urogenital tract, is closely followed by joint effusions, which themselves are sterile on culture.

Bacterial infection of bone (osteomyelitis) is sometimes associated with suppurative arthritis. Osteomyelitis may be the primary event, infection thence spreading to a joint cavity, whereas in other situations it is the synovial membrane which is first involved, organisms later invading neighbouring cartilage and bone.

As with many infectious diseases, the patterns of suppurative arthritis and osteomyelitis have changed greatly over the past 50 years, being modified by improving standards of social conditions, better individual health, and the introduction of antibiotics. Primary suppurative arthritis can occur at any age but is more frequent in the young, infection by bacteria–particularly the pus-forming organism *Staphylococcus aureus*–reaching the joint by way of the blood-stream from some other focus of infection such as a boil or dental abscess. Usually only one joint, such as the knee or hip, is involved, with high fever and acute pain and tenderness. Organisms can be isolated from culture of joint fluid or blood. With prompt diagnosis and antibiotic treatment the outlook is usually good, but this is not always the case when diagnosis is delayed or antibiotics are mishandled.

A number of special situations predispose to joint infection. The diseased synovial membrane in rheumatoid arthritis has a tendency to harbour invading micro-organisms and the presence of infection in an already inflamed joint may escape detection. Suppurative arthritis can occur in other debilitating diseases such as diabetes, and another problem is created by the increasing use, in many disorders, of drugs which modify the body's immune response. Rarely, infection can enter a joint by way of a needle introduced for diagnostic purposes, although of course this should never happen with proper sterile techniques.

Tuberculosis of bones, joints, and tendon sheaths, formerly a very common disease of childhood, is now much less frequent owing to the preventative measures which have been taken to control tuberculosis in our communities; when it does occur it can usually be effectively treated with the antibiotics which are today available. Tuberculosis is seen at any age and is not uncommon among some of the immigrant population of the United Kingdom.

Other special types of bacterial infective arthritis include those caused by the gonococcus, which is responsible for the venereal disease gonorrhoea (see Plate 20); the meningococcus, which is classically associated with meningitis; brucella, which cause brucellosis or undulant fever and salmonella and shigella, organisms causing enteric fever and dysentery. Arthritis produced by the last two groups of bacteria is usually of the reactive variety but these organisms can also invade joints directly.

Polyarthritis, usually benign and transient, is also found in association with certain types of viral infection, most commonly rubella (German measles), where joint pain and swelling occur in about 15 per cent of cases. Signs of arthritis usually come on for a few days after the rash, but they can precede it or indeed occur without any obvious rash at all, when the diagnosis is made on the basis of the presence of antibodies in the blood. Other viral infections in which polyarthritis can occur include infective hepatitis (where the joint symptoms usually disappear with the onset of jaundice), influenza, mumps, smallpox, and infectious mononucleosis (glandular fever). It should perhaps be emphasized that the viral arthritis of this type is a well-documented association of viral infection and arthritis; it should be distinguished from such disorders as rheumatoid arthritis (Chapter 3) or systemic lupus erythematosus (Chapter 10), where some form of underlying viral cause has been suggested but remains unproved.

We should also perhaps mention various types of fungal infection which can involve joints, very rarely it is true, but rather more frequently with today's use of immunosuppressive drugs; and the bacterial infection which can complicate operative joint replacement in conditions such as rheumatoid arthritis and osteoarthrosis. This is also rare, which is just as well because it can be a very serious complication indeed, often necessitating removal of the prosthesis.

Arthritis connected with skin diseases

Some disorders, while primarily involving the skin, also cause a transient arthritis. Common among these are erythema nodosum and Henoch-Schonlein purpura.

Erythema nodosum

Red, tender areas, slightly raised above the surface of the skin, appear on the fronts of the lower legs, occasionally elsewhere; they persist for a few days or weeks, then clearing up completely, though occasionally recurring. Erythema nodosum is an inflammatory condition, forming part of a response to one of several external agents such as infections (for example streptococcal, tuberculous) or drugs. It may also be associated with ulcerative colitis and a chronic inflammatory illness known as sarcoidosis.

Joint symptoms occur in about 75 per cent of cases. Pain and swelling involve a variable number of joints; the erythrocyte sedimentation rate is raised but there is no permanent joint damage. The diagnosis is easy enough because of the unique appearance of the skin lesions, but difficulties arise when the arthritis comes first, as it often does. It is sometimes then regarded as a rather acute form of rheumatoid arthritis and anxiety is felt, but erythema nodosum and its joint manifestations are in themselves benign and self-limiting.

Henoch–Schonlein purpura

This again is considered to be an immunological reaction to an external agent, such as infection of foods, though the agent is not usually identified. The term 'purpura' refers to a rash of small haemorrhagic spots in the skin, and in the Henoch–Schonlein variety this is accompanied by episodes of abdominal pain and a transient arthritis involving several joints, those of the lower limb predominating. The disease is mainly one of young children, but it is occasionally seen in adults. The rash and joint symptoms recover completely: rarely the condition is followed by chronic nephritis and kidney failure.

Arthritis connected with disorders of the blood

A number of haematological diseases can present with joint problems as part of their symptomatology, due to combinations of bleeding into the joint cavity (haemarthrosis), clotting in blood vessels, and other pathological processes. Most of them are rare: we should mention haemophilia, leukaemia, and the haemoglobinopathies.

Haemophilia

Haemophilia is one of the numerous blood disorders characterized by an abnormality of the clotting mechanism, in this case a deficiency of the coagulation protein Factor VIII. It is a sex-linked hereditary disease, the gene for its transmission, like that for colour-blindness, being carried on the X-chromosome in such a way that possession of the gene by a male results in expression of the disease, but by a female in the asymptomatic 'carrier' state. The sons of a haemophilic man (provided that he does not have a carrier wife) will be normal: his

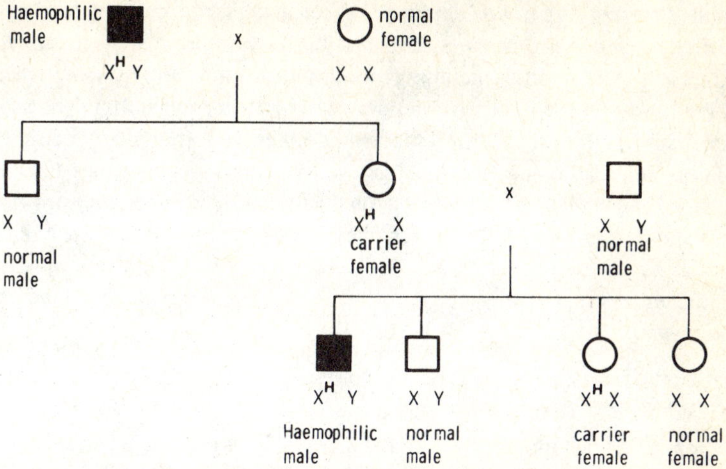

Fig. 6. Inheritance of haemophilia.

daughters will be carriers: and the son of a haemophilic carrier mother has a 50 per cent chance of possessing the gene (Fig. 6). The disease achieved notoriety during the last century as the gene worked its way through the inter-marrying Royal Houses of Europe.

Recurrent bleeding into joints is common, occurring after minor injuries or apparently spontaneously. The joint–usually the knee, elbow, or other large joint–becomes hot, red, swollen, and extremely painful, but this is relieved if Factor VIII is rapidly administered by intravenous injection. In patients with less than 2 per cent of the normal level of Factor VIII joint involvement tends to be especially severe, permanent damage resulting from recurrent bleeding, destruction of cartilage and bone, muscle contracture, and fusion of the bone ends (ankylosis) by fibrous tissue. Such deformities are nowadays preventable to a large extent by prompt treatment of acute episodes, and for already damaged joints reconstructive surgery can be undertaken under haematological control.

Leukaemia

Leukaemia is a condition in which the white cells of the blood proliferate in an uncontrolled fashion. The disease may be acute or chronic and different types are described according to the class of white cell affected. Deposits of the abnormal cells form in many organs and tissues of the body, including bone, periosteum, and synovial membrane, and there is also a tendency to haemorrhage. It is therefore not surprising that symptoms from bones and joints are common. These include pain, swelling, and joint effusion, sometimes haemorrhagic. Such features are often overshadowed by other more important effects of the disease, but when they appear at the onset of the illness they may present a diagnostic problem, especially in children, in whom leukaemia must always be considered as a rare cause of bone and joint pain.

Haemoglobinopathies

There are certain genetic abnormalities in the molecular structure of haemoglobin, the oxygen-carrying material in the red cell, which produce abnormalities in the shape of the cell with a consequent predisposition to thrombosis within the small blood vessels. Prominent among these is sickle-cell disease and its variants, where clotting of blood and obstruction of its flow in the vessels of the bone ends, particularly the heads of the femur (thigh-bone) and humerus (upper arm), lead to local death of bone tissue and acutely painful joints.

Sickle-cell disease occurs in Negro races: other haemoglobinopathies are found in Mediterranean and Eastern European peoples. Formerly seldom encountered in the United Kingdom, they are now familiar to physicians treating large numbers of immigrants or visitors to this country.

Injury

In Chapter 3 it was pointed out that the development of rheumatoid arthritis in susceptible persons was dependent to some extent on joint movement and could be exacerbated or precipitated by local injury, while in Chapter 6 we saw how osteoarthrosis could follow severe, prolonged, or recurrent trauma to a joint, and how hypermobile joints are specially vulnerable to trauma and to later development of osteoarthrosis.

Other forms of arthritis

Injury to a normal joint can produce synovitis with swelling due to effusion and synovial thickening. The injury may be external, as from a blow or fall, or internal, as when a knee is twisted playing football. Such a traumatic synovitis is specially liable to occur if the joint is already damaged by osteoarthrosis, when indeed a painful joint effusion can follow such minor degrees of injury as to have escaped notice. Provided there is no significant damage to bone or cartilage, traumatic synovitis usually clears up without any residual trouble.

Traumatic lesions of meniscal cartilages of the knee are common in young adult games-players. If the symptoms of pain and locking of the joint are persistent the damaged cartilage may need to be removed surgically.

Bone death (osteonecrosis)

Sickle-cell disease is not the only situation in which interruption of blood supply can cause local bone death, so-called avascular necrosis of bone, or osteonecrosis. Similar changes, with pain usually in the hip or shoulder, occur in such differing conditions as rheumatoid arthritis, systemic lupus erythematosus (Chapter 10), corticosteroid therapy, and alcoholism ('boozer's hip'), although their causative mechanisms are by no means well understood. Osteonecrosis also occurs in various forms in childhood ('osteochondritis'). An occupational type is known as Caisson disease, in which bubbles of nitrogen form in small blood vessels as a diver passes too rapidly from a high pressure to a lower one.

A special form of osteonecrosis, quite common in young adults, especially men, is known as osteochondritis dissecans. Here a single joint, usually the knee, becomes painful and swollen and X-ray shows that a fragment of cartilage with its underlying bone has become partially or completely separated (see Plate 21). Osteoarthrosis may follow in later years. Symptoms sometimes remit spontaneously but surgical intervention is often necessary to remove the loose fragment.

Charcot joints

Charcot was one of the great French neurologists of the last century, working at the famous Saltpêtrière Hospital in Paris. He recognized a remarkable form of arthritis which occurred in patients with a neurological disease called tabes dorsalis, which is a late stage (occurring many years after infection) of the venereal disease syphilis, caused by the organism *Spirochaeta pallida*. In Charcot's day syphilis was rampant and there was no effective treatment; tabetics presented a striking and common clinical picture.*

The Charcot (or neuropathic) joint, typically a single knee, is an extreme form of osteoarthrosis: relentless destruction of cartilage and bone is accompanied by effusion, massive bony outgrowths, and instability. The process is on the whole surprisingly painless, and indeed loss of pain sensation, which is normally a protective mechanism after minor degrees of injury, is thought to be an important factor permitting the progressive damage which occurs in a Charcot joint.

Today, syphilis is uncommon and easily treated in its early stages: medical students no longer sing about tabes, and rheumatologists rarely see a Charcot joint. Neuropathic arthropathy can, however, occasionally complicate other neurological disorders. For example, diabetes when accompanied by damage to the nerves may be associated with a neuropathic joint in the foot or ankle, and the same applies to a disease of the spinal cord called syringomyelia, although here the main disturbance of pain sensation is in the upper limbs and it is the shoulder which is usually involved.

Tumours

Tumours in or near joints are not common and their classification

*An old medical student's song, sung to the tune of the hymn 'The Church's one foundation', ran:

We are the three tabetics,
We've caught the spirochaete.
We haven't any knee jerks,
We walk on woolly feet.
Our pupils are eccentric,
They don't react to light.
Oh, give us some Salvarsan
To ease our sorry plight!

Salvarsan was the arsenical predecessor to penicillin.

is difficult, so that little need be said about them.

Pigmented villonodular synovitis is a special kind of synovial proliferation, in which the synovial membrane is dark brown in colour owing to the presence of iron. A heavily blood-stained effusion is present, usually in a single joint only.

The commonest malignant tumours found in bones or joints are secondary deposits from primary carcinoma elsewhere, especially the lung and breast. Primary malignant tumours of synovial membrane (synovioma) or bone (osteogenic sarcoma) show themselves as localized swellings. Multiple myeloma is a widespread malignant proliferation of plasma cells in bone marrow: not an uncommon condition, it must always be suspected when persistent bone pain, particularly back pain, develops in the elderly. Diagnosis is made by characteristic X-ray appearances, a raised erythrocyte sedimentation rate, blood protein changes, and the finding of excess plasma cells in the marrow.

10

Inflammatory disorders of connective tissue

The inflammatory disorders of connective tissue constitute a number of conditions—often rather ill-defined and of unknown cause—which in the past have been regarded as separate entities and having little in common with the rheumatic diseases as they were generally understood, but which now lie firmly within the province of the rheumatologist. This is for two main reasons.

In the first place, research over the past 30 years has shown that there is considerable overlap between this group of diseases and other rheumatic disorders with regard to serological abnormalities. Thus, rheumatoid factors which were described in Chapter 3 may also be found in these conditions, and the converse also applies: for example, antinuclear antibodies, a feature in particular of systemic lupus erythematosus, can also be detected in a proportion of patients with rheumatoid arthritis. Secondly, there is also a clinical overlap, again particularly with rheumatoid arthritis. Systemic lupus erythematosus patients may first consult their doctor with an inflammatory polyarthritis indistinguishable from that of rheumatoid disease; pericarditis and pleurisy can occur in rheumatoid arthritis, as can blood vessel changes indistinguishable from those of polyarteritis nodosa; and so on.

There are similar shared problems involving diagnosis and management. No apology is therefore needed for the introduction of this group of disorders into a book dealing with arthritis and rheumatism. It is conceded, however, that they are complex, difficult to understand, and relatively rare, so that our discussion of them can be fairly short. Four of them will be considered as individual diseases: polyarteritis nodosa, systemic lupus erythematosus, scleroderma, and dermatomyositis—though the reader will have already seen that their rigid classification into separate 'pigeon-holes' is not really possible and indeed this whole branch of medicine bristles with conceptual difficulties. These problems were appreciated as long ago as 1942 by the American physician Klemper and his colleagues, who coined the term 'collagen disease', a term which enjoyed a considerable vogue for some years, but which has now been rightly abandoned; with the exception of scleroderma collagen is not primarily involved and the use of the label 'collagen disease' has encouraged further diagnostic obfuscation in an area which is already murky enough.

Polyarteritis nodosa and other types of vasculitis

'Polyarteritis' means widespread inflammation of arteries, especially small arteries; 'nodosa' refers to the nodular inflammatory swellings of arteries (due to weakening of their walls) which were emphasized in early descriptions of the last century; 'vasculitis' means inflammation of any sort of blood vessel.

Polyarteritis nodosa is a disease of unknown cause with characteristic inflammatory changes in the walls of small and medium-sized arteries. Males are affected more frequently than females, the incidence rising with age, though occasionally the disease is seen in children.

Clinical symptoms and signs are due primarily to (1) widespread inflammatory changes and (2) obstruction of blood flow though affected vessels. Because a diversity of organs or tissues can be involved the manifestations vary greatly from case to case and diagnosis is often very difficult indeed. Against a background of signs of generalized inflammation–fever, weight loss, anaemia, and an elevated erythrocyte sedimentation rate–patients sooner or later show signs of malfunction in one or several systems of the body. For example, kidney involvement is common, with impaired excretory function and a rise in blood pressure, and other internal organs, including the heart and lungs, can also be affected. More superficial signs of the disease include abnormalities of movement and sensation in the limbs due to involvement of small arteries supplying the nerves; pain in muscles and joints; and a number of changes in the skin including ulceration and different kinds of rash. The diagnosis can be satisfactorily established by biopsy of an involved piece of tissue–removal of a minute portion for examination under the microscope.

The outlook is variable and unpredictable, depending on the severity of the inflammatory changes, their location, and duration. Thus mild involvement of, say, skin and muscle may cause relatively little trouble whereas more widespread polyarteritis in kidneys and other internal organs may have much more serious implications.

The basic causes of polyarteritis remain unknown, although some form of altered immunological reactivity, localized or generalized, is almost certainly implicated. Similar symptoms have been seen in patients with serum sickness (immunological reactions to animal serum given therapeutically) and in experimental animals. There is some support for the idea that human polyarteritis is due to circulating antigen–antibody complexes causing abnormalities in vessel walls in a genetically susceptible subject. The nature of such complexes is unknown: they could be viral. In this connection it is of interest that hepatitis-associated antigen has been identified in the serum and lesions of a proportion of patients with polyarteritis, suggesting that hepatitis virus can sometimes participate in causing the disease. The possible role of various types of infection was debated long before these recent observations. Polyarteritis has also been reported to follow the use of many different drugs. Retrospective data of this sort are difficult to interpret.

Signs of active inflammation are usually rapidly suppressed by corticosteroid hormones but the results of long-term treatment with steroids are more difficult to assess. Kidney failure with resultant high blood pressure are unfortunately often irreversible. Since there are grounds for supposing that immunological mechanisms are responsible for tissue damage in at least a proportion of cases of polyarteritis, the use of immunosuppressive agents such as azathioprine or cyclophosphamide appears logical but we have no clear idea of the value of such treatment.

There are various other types of vasculitis. Of particular interest to the rheumatologist are the blood vessel abnormalities which can be found in some patients with rheumatoid arthritis, to which brief reference was made in Chapter 3 (page 21). These lesions are of several varieties, ranging from a rather bland thickening of the internal coat of the artery, seen typically in the finger vessels, to widespread severe inflammatory changes, indistinguishable from those of classical polyarteritis nodosa. High levels of IgM rheumatoid factor are present in the blood and other extra-articular features, especially rheumatoid nodules, are often present.

Another quite common type of arterial inflammation is called 'temporal' or 'giant-cell' arteritis, because the temporal artery, which runs up to the scalp at the side of the face, becomes swollen and tender: under the microscope its walls can be seen to be infiltrated with inflammatory cells, including large cells with several nuclei called giant cells. Other arteries can also be affected. The usual onset is with pain in the head and face; among more serious effects are visual disturbance and blindness, so that prompt diagnosis and treatment (steroids are highly effective) are necessary. There is an intriguing association between temporal arteritis and polymyalgia rheumatica (Chapter 11, page 104).

Systemic lupus erythematosus

This is rather a mouthful and requires explanation. The word 'lupus', latin for wolf, has been used for about 400 years to signify a variety of scarring diseases of the skin and came to refer mainly to lupus vulgaris ('common lupus'), formerly a frequently seen form of tuberculosis affecting the skin. The facial rash of the disorder which we are about to consider was recognized over 100 years ago and was called lupus erythematosus on account of its redness. Viewed initially as purely a skin disease, it became increasingly recognized during the early years of the present century, largely owing to the clinical studies of William Osler, as a disorder sometimes involving many internal organs. The further adjective 'disseminated', or more recently 'systemic', was therefore added, and this is the term now used, usually abbreviated to SLE. By contrast, many patients do have a chronic skin disease only, usually without systemic features, and here the term 'discoid LE' is used.

The latest historical stage began 30 years ago with the discovery of the 'LE cell' and the recognition that this abnormal leucocyte was formed by the action of an antibody to cell nuclei present in the serum of patients with SLE. These and later discoveries have given us some idea about the mechanisms of this disease; they have also facilitated the diagnosis of mild forms, previously unrecognized, so that what was thought to be a rare and usually fatal disorder is now realized to be often relatively benign.

SLE is rare in males and is usually seen in young women. It is world-wide in distribution but appears to be more common in Negroes than whites.

As will be discussed below, the manifestations of SLE appear to be a direct consequence of immune reactions between different constituents of cell nuclei and corresponding auto-antibodies in the serum. Presumably the location of these reactions in the body are dependant on the exact nature and quantity of these antibodies, but knowledge about this is still incomplete. Like polyarteritis nodosa, therefore, the clinical features of SLE are highly variable, both in the sites involved and from time to time in the same patient.

Fever and other constitutional symptoms are usual and pain in the joints and muscles very common indeed. Joint swelling is similar to that found in rheumatoid arthritis and diagnosis between the two conditions may be difficult at first, although erosion of cartilage and bone does not occur in lupus arthritis to anything like the same extent as in rheumatoid disease. There are several different types of skin lesion, including the classical 'butterfly rash' over the cheeks and nose, sensitivity to sunlight, and hair loss. Vasculitis may be widespread, involving small blood vessels, and many patients complain of cold fingers. Any of the internal organs, such as the heart or lungs, can be affected, and the overall outlook depends to a large extent upon the degree and type of involvement of the kidneys and central nervous system.

Since SLE occurs predominantly in young women the question of pregnancy often arises. There is a high incidence of spontaneous miscarriage and the foetal death-rate is a little higher than normal but provided the heart and kidneys are functioning satisfactorily medical opinion would not be against a pregnancy.

Studies of the blood show the presence of numerous circulating antibodies, particularly those directed against nuclear constituents. The demonstration of antinuclear factors is a useful screening test, a negative test more or less excluding the diagnosis, but positive tests—though not as strong—are found in other conditions such as rheumatoid arthritis and a number of drug reactions. More specific for SLE are antibodies against a particular nuclear constituent known as native DNA (deoxyribose nucleic acid). There is good evidence that deposition of immune complexes of DNA and its antibody is responsible for much of the tissue damage in the kidneys, skin, and elsewhere. A rise in the level of DNA antibodies and a fall in serum complement (page 27) sometimes accompanies or precedes an exacerbation of kidney disease. Many other auto-antibodies have been found in patients with SLE, including rheumatoid factors.

Although this tells us a good deal about the mechanisms of tissue damage in SLE, the underlying causes of the disease, and the reasons for the development of this multiplicity of auto-antibodies, remain uncertain. There is no doubt that there is a radical disorder of normal immunological control with a disturbance of complex interrelationships between T lymphocytes and B lymphocytes (page 27). Research over the past few years has been exploring the possibility of a viral infection occurring in genetically susceptible individuals.

Mild cases require little in the way of treatment beyond the use of drugs such as aspirin to relieve pain and general advice about matters such as the avoidance of sunlight. Active disease, particularly with kidney or nervous system involvement, is a very different matter: corticosteroids, antimalarial drugs, immunosuppressive agents, and antibiotics to control the infections to which these patients are so susceptible all have a part to play.

Scleroderma (progressive systemic sclerosis)

In this whole difficult field of connective tissue disorders, where our knowledge of underlying causes is so unsatisfactory and our therapeutic ability is so limited, none is more mysterious than scleroderma. We really have no idea why the skin slowly tightens, the blood vessels become narrow, and deposits of calcium form in the subcutaneous tissue.

Scleroderma, which means 'hard skin', was described several hundred years ago. It is indeed predominantly a skin disorder, and like SLE was formerly regarded as being exclusively so. Later it became realized that there were sometimes important features in the internal body systems, emphasized by the South African physician Koetz when he coined the term 'progressive systemic sclerosis'.

There are two main components of this disorder. First, in the skin there is a low-grade inflammatory reaction followed by a progressive increase in the quantity of collagen, and secondly the internal lining of the blood vessels thickens and sometimes there are more acute inflammatory changes, for example in the kidneys. Other changes include deposition of calcified nodules under the skin, infiltration of muscle and synovial membrane with inflammatory cells, degeneration of the walls of the oesophagus (gullet), and fibrosis in lung and cardiac muscle.

The disease can start at any age but is commonest in adults, women being more frequently affected than men. The onset is very insidious with rigidity and tightening of the skin which becomes tethered to deeper structures. Initially only the fingers, hands, and feet are involved but the process may spread to the limbs, face, and trunk. It should nevertheless be emphasized that progression is not invariable and that spontaneous improvement occasionally happens. Along with the skin changes, and sometimes preceding them, the skin of the fingers becomes excessively pale, then blue, on exposure to cold (Raynaud's phenomenon). This deprivation of blood supply can progress to painful and distressing ulceration of the fingers with extrusion of subcutaneous calcific nodules. Other features present to a variable extent include synovitis in joints and tendon-sheaths, difficulty in swallowing, progressive shortness of breath if there is the lungs are affected, weight loss, and occasionally kidney failure with a raised blood pressure.

Overlap with other connective tissue disorders is sometimes seen, particularly with SLE and dermatomyositis, although the disease usually retains its own very distinctive features. Antinuclear antibodies occur in a proportion of cases, but they appear to be qualitatively different from those found in SLE and the presence of DNA antibodies is exceptional.

Polymyositis and dermatomyositis

Polymyositis is a term used to denote diffuse inflammation and weakness in voluntary muscles: when associated with a characteristic skin rash the condition is termed dermatomyositis. Here again attempts at classification are unsatisfactory.

Polymyositis can develop at any age and is rather commoner in females. The onset of weakness and pain in the muscles may be rapid or insidious, with varying degrees of disability, severe cases showing progressive involvement of the muscles of respiration. Later changes are those of muscle contracture and wasting.

The rash of dermatomyositis consists of reddish-purple discoloration of the eyelids, forehead, face, fingers, and sometimes elsewhere. Mild arthritis sometimes occurs and rarely the heart and lungs are involved, as in scleroderma.

Separate problems arise in children and in adults. In children, in addition to the skin and muscular changes, vasculitis is common, with sequels such as cold fingers and ulceration of the skin. Children also have a tendency to develop calcinosis—hard calcified deposits under the skin similar to those occurring in scleroderma, but much more extensive. Contractures are also much more of a problem in children. In adults, there is an unexplained association with cancer in between 10 and 20 per cent of cases, usually a carcinoma of lung, uterus, or ovary.

It has been claimed that lymphocytes from untreated patients have a direct toxic effect on muscle cell cultures, indicating a cell-mediated immunological abnormality (page 27); there is also evidence to suggest immune complex deposition as a cause of vasculitis. These conclusions should still be regarded as tentative and in any case underlying causes remain unknown.

Corticosteroids are often capable of suppressing disease activity, and where they are ineffective immunosuppressive drugs such as methotrexate or cyclophosphamide can be used. No drugs have been shown to influence the development of calcinosis. In adults, a careful search for malignancy is necessary.

11

Rheumatic disease that does not involve joints

It may have occurred to the reader, thumbing through the previous chapters, that many of the conditions described were rather rare and exotic, hardly conforming to his idea of 'rheumatism'. They are, in fact, all important rheumatic diseases, but, with the exception of minor degrees of osteoarthrosis, the average man or woman can reasonably expect to go through life without encountering any of them.

The average man or woman will, however, be extremely fortunate to escape some of the conditions to be described in this chapter, which will deal with a number of different rheumatic conditions in which joints are not primarily affected—'non-articular' disease. Some are uncommon, but others, such as disc injuries or inflammation of tendons or bursae after exercise or injury, are familiar to us all.

Polymyalgia rheumatica

This is a disorder of the elderly, of unknown cause, characterized by marked pain and stiffness of the shoulder and hip regions. Although in its typical form it is a striking and unmistakable syndrome, it often passes undiagnosed and is therefore the cause of considerable discomfort and disability. It is one of the commoner rheumatic diseases, being estimated to affect about 1 in 50 of the elderly population.

Its rather cumbersome name was introduced 20 years ago and is now generally accepted, although a number of others have been used. As was pointed out in Chapter 1, the term 'fibrositis' has been avoided in this book because, like 'rheumatism', it cannot be defined; there is little doubt that at least some of the patients who were previously labelled as having fibrositis were suffering from what we now call polymyalgia rheumatica. The same probably refers to the old name 'muscular rheumatism'.

The disease is about four times as common in women as in men, and usually occurs after the age of 60. Over the course of a few days or weeks, sometimes more quickly, increasingly severe pain develops in the neck, shoulders, upper arms, buttocks, and thighs. The pain is worse on movement so that it is difficult to walk briskly or climb stairs. A constant feature is severe morning stiffness lasting several hours, comparable to that occurring in rheumatoid arthritis, except that the joints are rarely swollen.

The erythrocyte sedimentation rate is almost invariably raised: apart from mild anaemia other laboratory tests are negative.

An interesting association is with temporal arteritis (page 99), although the nature of this association, like the actual causes of the two conditions, is unknown. About half of all patients with temporal arteritis go through an initial phase of polymyalgic symptoms; a rather smaller proportion of patients with polymyalgia develop features of temporal arteritis. Biopsy examination of temporal arteries may show inflammatory changes even in the absence of symptoms.

The condition responds dramatically to corticosteroid treatment, for example 15 mg of prednisolone daily, which is slowly reduced to a considerably lower maintainance dose, and it is often possible to withdraw the drug altogether over a period of months. The use of steroids is usually necessary because the condition does not respond well to other anti-inflammatory drugs (although these may be tried in the first place). Moreover, a suppressive dose of prednisolone safeguards against the chance that temporal arteritis, with its risk of sudden blindness, may also be present.

Back pain and disc injury

We have nearly all had back pain to a greater or lesser degree; it is the most common rheumatic symptom. It has been estimated that 2 per cent of the population go to their doctor every year because of backache, and Dr. Philip Wood, of the Arthritis and Rheumatism Council Field Unit, recently reported that in one year it led to 390 000 spells of incapacity and 13.2 million working days lost in this country. There is a clearly demonstrated association between back pain and heavy manual work, indicating the importance of environmental and occupational factors.

There are numerous causes of backache, which fall into several categories.

1 *Structural derangements.* The commonest and most important of these is prolapse of an intervertebral disc with damage to associated ligaments (the basic anatomy of vertebrae and discs was outlined in Chapter 2, page 18).
2 *Degenerative changes.* These include spondylosis (not to be confused with spondylitis), which consists of chronic degeneration and narrowing of the intervertebral discs with bony outgrowths (osteophytes) projecting from the vertebral margins, and osteoarthrosis involving the small joints at the back of the vertebrae.
3 *Developmental abnormalities*, such as narrowing of the spinal canal (which transmits the spinal cord) and spondylolisthesis, a congenital displacement of the vertebrae.
4 *Ankylosing spondylitis* and allied conditions (Chapter 5).
5 *Infections* of the vertebrae, discs, or related structures, for example tuberculous, staphylococcal, or salmonella infections.
6 *Tumours*, either primary growths or secondary deposits in the vertebrae from primary carcinomas of lung, breast, or prostate gland: also multiple myeloma (Chapter 9, page 95).
7 *Other types of bone disorder*, such as metabolic bone disease (Chapter 8, page 77); Paget's disease of bone.
8 *Referred back pain* from other internal structures, for example from duodenal ulcer or carcinoma of the pancreas.

I shall not discuss this list in any detail, but two general points may be made. In the first place, the list of causes of backache (which is by no means complete) is a long one and contains a number of serious medical conditions. A busy rheumatology clinic, dealing with several hundred patients with backache every year, will encounter among them about half a dozen with tumours or infections requiring urgent investigation and treatment. Medical advice should therefore always be sought for persistent back pain.

Secondly, the conditions listed are all amenable to more or less precise identification, but doctors see many patients with chronic back pain where it is not possible to reach a definitive diagnosis. It is important to recognize these areas where we are as yet ignorant. Professor Malcolm Jayson, who has studied back pain extensively, advises the use of the phrase 'non-specific back pain' for such cases. Whether the term is the right one or not is debatable–after all, the cause of the pain in any one patient may be specific enough, it is just that we do not know what it is–but we should certainly resist the temptation to use quasi-precise terms such as 'lumbo-sacral strain' which lack either a pathological basis or a satisfactory clinical description.

A lesion of one or more intervertebral discs in the lumbar region is the commonest cause of low back pain. Material from the soft, pulpy centre of the disc herniates through the fibrous ring around it to press on associated structures, important among which are pain-sensitive ligaments and nerve-roots emerging from the spinal canal to passing close behind the discs. Pain may be sudden in onset, situated in the back alone ('lumbago') or radiating down one or both lower limbs ('sciatica'), often coming on during some stressful movement of the trunk. Alternatively it may commence gradually with no obvious precipitating factor. The examining physician will find limitation of spinal movement and perhaps abnormal neurological signs if the protruding disc is pressing on nerve roots.

It is advisable for the patient to rest in bed, on a firmly supported mattress, until the pain has subsided, and indeed its severity may force him to do so. Powerful analgesics such as pethidine may be necessary at first, but in most cases the pain settles in a few days, or perhaps weeks, as the extruded portion of disc scars and shrinks. (Contrary to popular conception, the disc does not pop in and out of place!).

As the patient becomes mobilized he should wear a strong, properly fitted lumbar corset with steel braces in the back for some months: apart from the support provided it serves as a reminder against sudden unwise movements of the trunk as the damaged disc continues to heal. Advice is necessary about protecting the spine during lifting and bending; movement should take place at the hips and knees rather than by flexing the back. As work is resumed attention must be paid to any occupational factors which may have contributed to the disorder. In the case of a worker in heavy industry this may be a counsel of perfection, but it may be possible to modify a job in a helpful way. In sedentary occupations proper support of the low back in the seated position is important; this includes back supports for car seats.

The patient may reasonably hope to recover completely and return to a full active life, but any person who has had a disc injury is at some risk of a recurrence, and a minority of individuals are unfortunate enough to develop chronic persistent back pain.

Physiotherapy may be helpful but its place is limited. Warmth is comforting and it is customary to prescribe 'extension exercises'. The value of these is doubtful and I have seen them produce a smart recurrence of lumbar disc pain in a patient who up to that time had been convalescing satisfactorily. Certainly the approach to such gymnastics should be very cautious. Intermittent spinal traction is also employed, but again its value has never been demonstrated in any form of controlled trial.

Much has been written about spinal manipulation and the numerous different techniques used for this. It has been claimed that such techniques can reduce the size of a disc herniation and very occasionally patients report dramatic improvement of pain following the procedure. Controlled trials are difficult to organize in this situation where the tendency is in any case towards spontaneous improvement, but such trials as have been conducted have failed to show any overall advantage from this form of treatment. Certainly the torn, inflamed intervertebral disc would normally be expected to heal more readily and naturally under conditions of rest than while subjected to forcible movements which might produce yet further damage.

In recent years a method has been developed of injecting local anaesthetic with steroid, contained in a large volume of salt solution, into the space surrounding the spinal cord (extradural injection), and this has been reported to be effective in relieving pain, as has injection of a protein-destroying enzyme into the prolapsed portion of disc itself. General experience of these procedures remains limited, but it is likely that they will be of help in a few isolated cases only. Interest has also been revived in the ancient Chinese technique of acupuncture, in which fine needles are inserted into the skin. Again, therapeutic trials are lacking and the physiological principles by which acupuncture might be effective in relieving pain—other than by psychological auto-suggestion—are by no means clear.

It is sometimes necessary to consider surgical removal of a herniated disc, before which it is usual to carry out further investigations—for example, the special X-ray procedure known as myelography—to determine precisely the site and extent of the damage. The indications for surgery are (1) intractable pain not responding to other forms of treatment, and (2) the presence or persistence of significant neurological abnormalities such as weakness or sensory loss. With carefully selected patients surgery is successful in about 80 per cent of cases.

Many of these considerations about lumber disc lesions apply also to disc herniation in the neck or cervical region, the other common site. Again the onset may be gradual or sudden, sometimes following trauma such as a 'whiplash' car injury, and pain may be localized to the head and neck or radiate down one or both arms as a result of nerve root pressure. The principles of treatment are similar: rest is indicated for severe cases and many different types of collar have been designed to immobilize the neck. In the thoracic region, the intervertebral discs are thinner than in the lumbar and cervical regions, because less movement takes place between the thoracic vertebrae, and disc lesions here are rare.

Our knowledge of back pain is still all too imprecise. Our ignorance of pathology and treatment of organic lesions is complicated by the unfortunate fact that chronic back pain is a common expression of neurosis.

Bursitis

A bursa is a closed, slit-like cavity, lined with synovial membrane, found in any part of the body where movement occurs—for example, between the skin and underlying bony prominences such as the elbow or knee, or between different muscle planes. Bursae are lubricated by synovial fluid, their walls gliding freely, thus serving to facilitate the play of one neighbouring structure upon another. Bursae in the neighbourhood of a joint may be continuous with the cavity of the joint through an aperture in the capsular ligament; there are several important bursae, for example, in relation to the shoulder and knee joints.

Bursae become inflamed when they are subjected to excessive or unusual movement. This condition of *bursitis* is extremely common and is responsible for many aches and pains which come and go throughout our lives. Bursitis can occur in many different sites, some of them classically related to the occupations of yesterday—for example, weaver's bottom, housemaid's knee, and policeman's heel (the latter referring to an age when the policeman on his beat was less mechanized than his modern counterpart). Occasionally the inflammation in the bursal cavity is associated with deposition of calcium salts, which show up on X-rays—*calcific bursitis*.

An attack of bursitis often recovers with rest: failing this a local injection of corticosteroid hormone, such as prednisolone, will usually deal with it.

Tenosynovitis

Many tendons are lined by a sheath of synovial membrane which facilitates their movement in a manner similar to that in which bursae ease the movement of one structure upon another. Inflammation of synovial membrane in this situation is called *tenosynovitis*. Tenosynovitis can be part of a general disease—for example rheumatoid arthritis, where the tendons in the palm of the hand are especially liable to be involved, or psoriatic arthritis. Often, like bursitis, tenosynovitis occurs simply as a result of local injury or strain, and is treated in a similar fashion. The tendon which extends the thumb, as it passes over the wrist, is particularly susceptible.

Tendinitis

Rather than the tendon sheath, a tendon itself may be the site of disease, as when rheumatoid nodules (Chapter 3, page 21) form in the tendons, which can lead to rupture. Localized tendinitis, often due to minor injuries or unknown causes, is especially liable to occur in some of the tendons related to the shoulder joint, such as one of the tendinous origins of the biceps muscle, or the tendon of a muscle called supraspinatus, where calcium deposition is often seen on X-ray. The course of tendinitis is variable but symptoms usually subside spontaneously, being helped by such measures as rest and local injection of a steroid hormone.

Tenoperiosteal lesions

The junctions of tendons or muscles to bone are susceptible to minor damage because of muscle pull. The commonest situation for this is where the extensor muscles of the wrist, lying on the back of the forearm, arise by a common tendon from the bony knob on the outside of the elbow. This is commonly known as 'tennis elbow' because it characteristically follows the strain imposed by backhand strokes at tennis; but it can also follow many other types of muscular activity, often unrecognized as being traumatic. Movements of the elbow and gripping movements of the hand are painful and the outer side of the elbow is tender. Recovery often occurs naturally but this can usually be accomplished immediately by an injection of local anaesthetic mixed with a corticosteroid. 'Golfer's elbow' is a similar lesion on the inner side of the elbow.

Some other soft-tissue problems

'Frozen shoulder' is a common complaint in which movement at the shoulder is limited and painful, not because of disease in the actual joint itself, but because of inflammatory or adhesive changes in the surrounding tissue. For this reason it is sometimes referred to as 'pericapsulitis'. Pain and stiffness develop slowly over a period of weeks or months, only to recover again equally slowly. Because spontaneous recovery is the rule, treatment is best restricted to conservative physiotherapy such as warmth and gentle assisted exercises. Steroid injections may help, but rather unpredictably. It has to be admitted that occasional intractable cases have been seen to recover immediately following sudden movement or manipulation, but such manoeuvres are seldom necessary or indicated, being not entirely free from the risk of causing further damage or even fractures.

Sometimes a frozen shoulder is part of the curious 'shoulder-hand syndrome', where limitation of shoulder movement is accompanied by changes in the hand on the same side–at first pain, warmth, and swelling, subsequently coldness and contractures of the fingers. If the condition occurs on both sides it can easily be mistaken for rheumatoid arthritis.

These shoulder syndromes may arise on their own, or sometimes they are associated with conditions causing pain or immobilization in the region–for example following coronary thrombosis, shingles, a stroke with paralysis on the affected side, or local injury. They also appear more liable to occur during periods of depression or anxiety.

A condition frequently involving the wrist and hand is the so-called 'carpal tunnel syndrome', in which one of the nerves supplying the hand (the median nerve) becomes compressed as it passes through the carpal tunnel in the wrist. The characteristic symptoms are tingling in the thumb, index, and middle fingers, often waking the patient at night. Sometimes secondary to an underlying condition such as rheumatoid arthritis, the carpal tunnel syndrome also occurs in pregnancy and in other situations when the body retains fluid; but usually its cause is uncertain. It responds to a local injection of steroid or to a very simple operation which releases the median nerve.

'Dupuytren's contracture' is the name given to a contracture of the subcutaneous tissue of the palm of the hand leading to a flexion deformity of the fingers. Its cause is unknown: there is sometimes an association with epilepsy or alcoholism though it often occurs in the absence of these associations. The only effective remedy lies in plastic surgery.

The strong thick tissues running forward from the heel under the sole of the foot may become painful and inflamed, especially at their origin of attachment to the heel-bone. Sometimes this lesion is due to trauma whereas in other cases it may be part of a generalized rheumatic disease, particularly ankylosing spondylitis or Reiter's syndrome (Chapter 5). Local steroid injections are usually effective.

The foot is well-known to be susceptible to a number of other minor but very troublesome and painful conditions such as hallux valgus (a sideways deviation of the great toe often associated with an overlying bunion) and other orthopaedic deformities of the arches of the feet and the bones and ligaments which form them.

There are numerous problems which contribute to the painful foot. By far the main culprit is faulty footwear. This starts with children of both sexes continuing to wear shoes a size or two too small for them. After this, however, boys and young men wear shoes which on the whole perform the protective function for which they were originally designed, whereas girls and young women (and old women) proceed to ruin their feet with high heels, which thrust the weight of the body on to the front of the feet, and pointed shoes, which finish things off by packing the toes together like a bunch of radishes. It is easy to understand why most of our middle-aged women have painful, deformed, and ugly feet, even when the rest of their anatomy is reasonably presentable. One might have hoped that the younger generation, with their more relaxed attitude to life in general, would avoid these difficulties, but as yet there are no clear signs of this, and our chiropodists, orthopaedic surgeons, and surgical appliance officers are not likely to lack work on this count for a long time yet.

12

Conclusion

So ends our survey of the rheumatic diseases. Some may have found it incomplete, as of course it is. No doubt the scientifically minded reader would have liked to learn more about basic principles of immunology or biochemistry and their important applications to this field of medicine. Others, on the other hand, might have preferred to read details of cider vinegar, homeopathy, copper bangles, the green-lipped mussel and other remedies.

The aim of the book has not been to cover everything–least of all to write a text-book–but rather to convey an idea of the multiplicity of rheumatic diseases and our current state of knowledge–and ignorance–about the more important of them. While the medical profession needs no reminding that our understanding of the causes and treatment of many of these disorders is imperfect, it should not be forgotten that others no longer present the same threat to health and longevity that they did only a relatively short time ago. Much is known about the causation of rheumatic fever and this dreadful disease of children has become a rarity in our developed countries (although admittedly this is owing rather to sociological than medical progress). Many of the underlying biochemical mechanisms of gout have been clarified and what was formerly a most painful and crippling disorder now yields readily to correct drug treatment. Antibiotics have dramatically changed the outlook in bacterial infections of joints and bones and no longer are children immobilized for months or years with their tuberculous hips or knees. The prognosis has also become considerably improved in the life-threatening inflammatory disorders of connective tissue.

On the other hand, knowledge of basic causes of rheumatoid arthritis and osteoarthrosis remains negligible. Although intense research has clarified some of the pathological processes taking place and standards of diagnosis and management have improved enormously, we have no concept of curative treatment or prevention, a goal which seems unlikely to be achieved for some years to come.

Organizations concerned with the rheumatic diseases

It may be useful to list some of the national societies and organizations which are concerned with the rheumatic diseases. These bodies will be pleased to offer advice, information and assistance.

Readers will, however, appreciate that such enquiries can be dealt with only in general terms. Individual patient care is the responsibility of the family doctor and the specialist or paramedical services at his disposal.

Arthritis and Rheumatism Council for Research
Faraday House, 8–10 Charing Cross Road
London WC2H 0HN (Tel. 01–240 0871)

Back Pain Association
Grundy House, Somerset Road
Teddington
Middlesex TW11 8TD (Tel. 01–977 1171)

British Lupus Society
(Contact through British Rheumatism and Arthritis Association)
6 Grosvenor Crescent
London SW1X 7ER (Tel. 01–235 0902)

British Red Cross Society
9 Grosvenor Crescent
London SW1X 7EJ (Tel. 01–235 5454)

British Rheumatism and Arthritis Association
6 Grosvenor Crescent
London SW1X 7ER (Tel. 01–235 0902)

Disabled Drivers' Association
Central Office
Ashwellthorpe Hall
Ashwellthorpe, Norwich NR16 1EX (Tel. Fundenhall (code 050–841) 449)

Disabled Drivers' Motor Club
9 Park Parade
Gunnersbury Avenue, London W3 9BD (Tel. 01–993 6454)

The Horder Centre for Arthritics
Crowborough
Sussex TN6 1XP (Tel. 08926 4141)

Arthritis and Rheumatism

National Ankylosing Spondylitis Society
31 Newcombe Road
Westbury on Trym
Bristol BS9 3QS (Tel. 0272 629846)

The Royal Association for Disability and Rehabilitation
25 Mortimer Street
London W1N 8AB (Tel. 01–637 5400)

Organizations in the United States

American Rheumatism Association
Arthritis Foundation
3400 Peachtree Road, N.E.
Atlanta, Georgia 30326 (Tel. (404) 266-0795)

Institute for Research of Rheumatic Diseases
Box 955, Ansonia Station
New York, New York 10023 (Tel. (212) 595-1368)

National Institute of Arthritis, Metabolism and Digestive Diseases
National Institutes of Health
Bethesda, Maryland 20205 (Tel. (301) 496-3583)

Glossary of terms

Analgesic: A pain-relieving drug.

Ankylosis: Fixation of a joint by disease.

Annulus fibrosus: The fibrous outer part of the intervertebral disc.

Antibody: A substance produced by the body to combine with a specific antigen.

Antigen: A substance capable of exciting an immunological response.

Arthrodesis: Surgical fixation of a joint.

Arthroplasty: Any form of surgical procedure which repairs a joint.

Autoimmunity: An abnormal immune reaction directed against a component of the host's own body tissue.

Bursa: A sac, other than a joint, which lies between moving parts of the body and which is lined by synovial membrane.

Bursitis: Inflammation of a bursa.

Cell-mediated immunity: A term referring to a type of immunological reaction in which antigen reacts directly with lymphocytes without the production of classical antibody.

Chondrocytes: Cells which make cartilage.

Chromosomes: Structures within cell nuclei which carry genes, the determinants of hereditary constitution.

Collagen: One of the main types of fibre of connective tissue.

Complement: A collective name for a number of proteins which are formed in sequence during some types of antigen–antibody reaction. Complement becomes incorporated in the antigen–antibody complex and can cause tissue damage and inflammation.

Connective tissue: The framework of the body, including bone, ligaments, cartilage, and less specialized 'packing material'.

Corticosteroid: *see* Steroids.

DNA: Deoxyribose nucleic acid. An important constituent of cell nuclei, antibodies to which are a feature of SLE.

Effusion: An excessive collection of fluid in a synovial joint (or any other body cavity).

Enzymes: Substances which accelerate specific organic chemical reactions in the body

Epidemiology: The study of health and disease in communities.

Erosion: Destruction of cartilage and bone by pannus.

Glossary

Erthrocyte sedimentation rate (e.s.r.): A laboratory test of inflammation, in which the rate of fall of red cells in a column of blood is measured.

Fibrocartilage: Cartilage containing dense fibrous bundles, forming an important part of such structures as intervertebral discs.

Flexion contracture: A state of permanent bending at a joint due to contraction of the strong flexor muscles. It occurs in various forms of arthritis, also in diseases of muscles and nerves.

Ground substance: Biological material which lies between cells and fibres of connective tissue.

Histocompatibility antigen: Antigens situated on the surface of lymphocytes and other cells which are responsible for rejection by the host of a graft from another person or animal of the same species. Histocompatibility antigens (also known as HLA or Human Leucocyte Antigens) of a particular type are sometimes associated with certain diseases, the most striking example being the association of HLA B27 with ankylosing spondylitis.

HLA B27: *see* Histocompatibility antigen.

Hyaline cartilage: Cartilage which exists as a layer over the surface of bone where it forms a synovial joint.

Hyperuricaemia: An excess of uric acid in the blood and tissues.

IgG: *see* Immunoglobulins.

IgM: *see* Immunoglobulins.

Immunoglobulins: Special proteins in the blood which form antibodies. There are five main classes (IgG, IgM, IgA, IgD, and IgE) which have different molecular structures and biological activities. IgG immunoglobulin acts as an antigen to IgM rheumatoid factor.

Immunology: The science of the body's defence system against infection, and its abnormalities.

Immunosuppression: Suppression of the immune response by drugs or other methods.

Intervertebral disc: Cartilagenous plates lying between the bones of the back (vertebrae).

Lesion: Any localized abnormality in a tissue or organ produced by injury or disease.

Lymphocyte: An immunologically active cell concerned with the production of antibody (B lymphocytes) or with cell-mediated immunity (T lymphocytes).

Matrix: Any type of biological material lying between the cells of the body.

Meniscus: A crescent-shaped piece of fibrocartilage lying within some joints, notably the knee.

Mucous membrane: A fluid-secreting membrane, for example that which lines the intestine.

Nucleus pulposus: The central soft part of the intervertebral disc.

Osteophyte: Outgrowths of bone from the edge of a joint, found in osteoarthrosis.

Glossary

Pannus: The inflamed swollen synovial membrane of rheumatoid arthritis.

Phagocytosis: Engulfing of foreign particles by cells.

Plasma: The fluid component of blood (as opposed to the blood cells).

Plasma cell: An antibody-producing cell derived from a lymphocyte.

Prolapse: A slipping out of place.

Prosthesis: An artificial joint inserted surgically.

Proteoglycan: The principal substance making up the ground substance of connective tissue.

Psoriasis: A common skin disorder producing red scaly areas, sometimes associated with arthritis.

Rehabilitation: The whole process of restoring a disabled person to a normal life.

Rheumatoid factor: Large molecular weight protein, mostly in IgM fraction, reacting with IgG immunoglobulin in rheumatoid arthritis.

Sacro-iliac joints: The joints between the base of the spine and the pelvic bones.

Sclerosis: Hardening (used, for example, to apply to arteries, bone, etc).

Seronegative arthritis: Inflammatory arthritis without the presence of rheumatoid factor.

Seropositive arthritis: Rheumatoid arthritis with the presence of rheumatoid factor.

Serum: Fluid obtainable from blood after it has clotted.

SLE: Systemic lupus erythematosus. An inflammatory disorder of connective tissue characterized by the presence of antibodies against various constituents of cell nuclei.

Steroids: A group of hormones, of which cortisone was the first to be used, with a dramatic anti-inflammatory effect.

Synarthrosis: Union between bones without a joint cavity.

Synovectomy: Surgical removal of the synovial membrane.

Synovial cells: Cells of the synovial membrane.

Synovial fluid: Fluid lying within a synovial joint.

Synovial joint: The mobile type of joint with a joint 'cavity'.

Synovial membrane: The membrane which lines the cavity of a synovial joint, tendon-sheath, or bursa.

Synovitis: Any form of inflammation of the synovial membrane.

Tenosynovitis: Inflammation of a tendon-sheath.

Tophus: A solid deposit of sodium urate.

Trauma: Injury.

Uric acid: A product of metabolism, excess of which can lead to gout. Deposition in the joints and elsewhere is in the form of the sodium salt (sodium urate).

Vasculitis: Inflammation of blood vessels.

Index

Index

Index